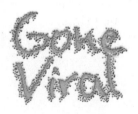

Frank Bowden graduated from the University of Melbourne in 1983 and undertook his basic physician training at St Vincent's Hospital in Fitzroy. He completed advanced training in infectious diseases at Fairfield Hospital in Melbourne at the height of the HIV epidemic. In the 1990s Frank Bowden worked as a clinician, researcher, administrator and public health physician in Darwin in his role as co-ordinator of the AIDS and STD programs for the Northern Territory. After a year in Oxford studying the mathematical modelling of infectious diseases he moved to Canberra in 1999, where he is foundation Professor of Medicine at the Australian National University Medical School and director of the Canberra Sexual Health Centre. Frank Bowden has been an adviser to the Australian government on HIV and sexually transmitted infections. He has edited a book on HIV, written chapters for several textbooks and has published over a hundred scientific articles. He is a board member of the One Disease at a Time Foundation.

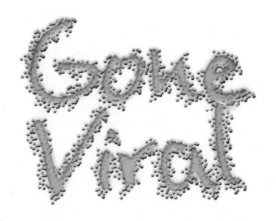

Gone Viral

The germs that
share our lives

FRANK BOWDEN

NEWSOUTH

To my mother, Joan, who was frightened of germs.
To my father, Kevin, who wasn't.

A NewSouth book

Published by
University of New South Wales Press Ltd
University of New South Wales
Sydney NSW 2052
AUSTRALIA
www.unswpress.com.au

© Francis Joseph Bowden 2011
First published 2011

10 9 8 7 6 5 4 3 2 1

National Library of Australia
Cataloguing-in-Publication entry
  Author: Bowden, Frank
  Title: Gone viral: the germs that share our lives, by Frank Bowden.
  ISBN: 978 174223 273 7 (pbk.)
  Subjects: Communicable diseases – Case studies.
          Public health – Social aspects – Case studies.
          AIDS (Disease) – Social aspects – Case studies.
  Dewey Number: 616.9

Design Josephine Pajor-Markus
Cover Nada Backovic Design, image courtesy of photolibrary
Printer Ligare

This book is printed on paper using fibre supplied from plantation or sustainably managed forests.

Contents

Author's note

Writing about your patients is a risky business for a doctor. The safest option is not to, and keep the things you have learnt to yourself. If you teach as well as practise medicine, then a select group of students may benefit from hearing about your experience in the consultation room, the operating theatre and the hospital ward. The next safest option is to record things as a novel and to include a disclaimer that (wink, wink) all of the characters are fictitious and bear no resemblance, and so on. Most controversially, a doctor may write openly and frankly about patients after they have died – Lord Moran was severely criticised for doing just that after the death of his most famous patient, Winston Churchill. (But what an insight this gave us into the effect that the illnesses suffered by one of the main protagonists of modern history had upon his decisions and actions.)

In writing this book I have tried to chart a course that provides the reader with an informative and, I hope, entertaining read while respecting and protecting the privacy of the patients that I have treated, regardless of the nature of the interactions I have had with them. The details of a consultation held in the middle of a busy ward should be no less confidential than one that takes place in a sexual health clinic. To ensure this confidentiality I have had to change a few crucial details in most stories – sometimes it will be the patient's age or profession, sometimes their gender. At times I have fiddled a little with the chronology, except when it is central to the context of the story.

Despite the myriad of combinations and permutations of human behaviour, and of the manifestations of disease, there is, thankfully for the learner, a smaller number of recurring patterns and themes that emerge in clinical practice. So while I hope that all of the vignettes that I have painted will sound familiar, no reader should assume that the patients depicted point to specific individuals. I am sad to say that many of the young patients that I describe in this book died during the first decade of the HIV epidemic and I wish that I could more openly memorialise them.

I have taken a slightly different line with colleagues and acquaintances, where my interactions have not been bound by the ethics of the doctor–patient relationship. I have avoided using the names of a few, occasionally to protect them, sometimes to protect me.

Introduction

My mother had scarlet fever as a young girl. She lived through epidemics of whooping cough, measles and polio, and her personal experience made her quite neurotic about germs. She would make me wash my hands if I handled money – coins or notes, it didn't matter. She was going to cancel my brother's tenth birthday party because he had a cold, and she wouldn't let him blow out the candles on the cake because of the risk of 'viral icing contamination', until my godmother saved the day by cutting out a protective paper 'condom' for the cake so just the tops of the candles showed. My mother made me put toilet paper on any 'foreign' toilet seat before I sat on it, and I even had to float a layer of tissue on the water in the bowl at home to minimise the risk of a splash on to my naked bottom. There was no three second rule in our household – if any part of a tea towel touched the floor for even an instant it was immediately dispatched to the washing machine. A cracked cup went straight in the bin because of the risk of catching TB from it (I have absolutely no idea where that one came from). Dogs were walking culture media to my mum – a pat followed by hand-washing was acceptable, but if I was licked on the face she would try to dab out the slobber from my mouth with her handkerchief.

We never ate rabbit in our household because mum knew that they all had myxomatosis. To my father's protests she would simply reply, 'If it can kill those poor little bunnies … ' Food was never reheated in the oven, and a can that had a dint in it would be thrown away, as it was well known, she told me, that you could get ptomaine poisoning – whatever that was – from such damaged containers. Our meals were never left uncovered for even a moment in case a fly landed and unloaded its deadly payload of detritus. In fact, my mum may have been the person that the copywriters had in mind when they invented Louie the Fly – our house was more likely to smell of Mortein than Chanel No. 5.

When I came home from a game of football during the winter she would run a bath and add two capfuls of Dettol to sterilise any residual dirt from the playing field that might be clinging to me. Her favourite antiseptic was acriflavine, a yellow liquid which she carefully applied to even the most minor of our cuts and abrasions, all of which would be carefully covered by a plastic band-aid. (I haven't seen a bottle of acriflavine for years. Derived from coal tar, this topical antiseptic was discovered by Paul Ehrlich in 1912 – around the same time he discovered Salvarsan, the first effective antimicrobial agent for syphilis.)

Contagion was, by far, highest on her list of worries. For although she lived in constant fear of me 'catching something', she would let me, as a scrawny 10 year old with a school bag that weighed more than I did, catch a bus from our home in Ashwood to Box Hill station, then a train to Camberwell and finally walk a kilometre to my school.

I was a boy in a bubble of maternal microbiological anxiety and I often wonder how my mother would have coped if she knew that I grew up to be an infectious diseases specialist. (There is no such thing as coincidence, a friend once told me, alluding to the deep psychological forces which he believed had pushed me in that particular vocational direction.)

My mum was at the far end of the germ-phobic spectrum, but most members of her generation possessed a healthy reverence for micro-organisms, based on things that they had seen with their own eyes. They had parents who had succumbed to pneumonia, friends who had died after a simple cut had turned into an abscess and then to 'blood-poisoning'. My father, who wasn't frightened of many things, always told me that I must never pick a pimple on my face if it was above the level of my upper lip. He didn't know why, he just knew that something bad could happen if you did (and he was right: infections on the upper part of the face can spread to a vein that traverses the brain, causing meningitis and stroke). When he was a teenager, his mother lived in fear of him contracting polio during the 1938 epidemic in Melbourne – the year that they closed the schools and came close to putting barricades on the bridges over the Yarra. My grandparents' generation embraced antibiotics and vaccinations as soon as they became available because they could see a direct benefit – they didn't need to imagine what a child with whooping cough or diphtheria looked like, they had lived it.

This book is written for people who haven't had the chance to see for themselves the harm that bacteria and viruses can inflict on human beings. As a doctor who trained to be an infectious diseases physician, not a microbiologist, I am much more interested in the way that germs affect the humans that they infect than in the germ itself. It's not that I don't like germs – I am rather attached to them actually, and they to me – but my time spent in a laboratory taught me that I was more comfortable by the bedside than at the benchtop.

The relationship between humans and pathogens is one of the most fascinating stories of evolution. Our species had to evolve in a world that was swarming with invisible microorganisms that would kill us if we had not developed an effective immune system. We are, you see, literally outnumbered. There were, at last count, 750 trillion (that's 750 million million) bacteria in the average human gut, but there are only about 100 trillion cells in the human body. The protective adaptations that have occurred over millions of years can be rapidly subverted by social changes that human societies can make in the space of a generation. New infectious diseases emerge as a result of alterations in the way humans congregate in cities and towns and how they interact with each other, as much as by modifications of the genetic structure of bacteria and viruses that make them more virulent or contagious.

The book is divided into 15 chapters, each based on an individual micro-organism or 'bug', as we infectious diseases people call them in a perhaps over-familiar way. There are five viruses, seven bacteria, two fungi and a parasite – all potential villains except for one of the fungi. Many readers will be directly or indirectly acquainted with some of them. They include HIV, influenza viruses and SARS – all of which have in recent times rivalled the ability of slightly more complex life-forms, such as politicians, movie stars and sportspeople, to hog the media spotlight. Other bugs, though, will probably be unfamiliar: one chapter deals with a parasite that infects at least 200 million people worldwide, but you would be hard pressed to find a non-medical person in Australia who could tell you much about it.

There are several themes that run through the book and I have tried to use specific examples of diseases to illustrate general concepts. Perhaps the prevailing theme is that the interventions that led to the control of infectious diseases have been victims of their own success – the improvements in sanitation and housing that came with prosperity, the development of vaccines, and the discovery of antibacterial and antiviral agents changed the face of medicine in the 20th century. In the developed world, infectious diseases receded as cancer, heart disease and chronic diseases took over. Diseases which are now only seen by specialists like me (and even then only rarely) are usually invisible to the general population, and the relationship between an intervention and the disappearance of a disease is often not appreciated. For those of us who have treated children and adults with life-threatening infections that could have been avoided by immunisation, it is very hard to remain calm in the face of widespread anti-scientific, anti-vaccination advocacy.

Furthermore, the current generation of health professionals seems to have suffered a collective memory loss about the need for infection control. This amnesia has created a modern health system that confuses our current habits with principles. I have tried to explain why this might be, and to outline the potential remedies.

Bacterial resistance began the day the first antimicrobial agents were used in humans. Sixty years later some authorities are arguing that the Age of Antibiotics will soon be over. I don't question the plausibility of these predictions, but a preoccupation with resistant bacteria (often referred to as superbugs) can distract us from the fact that most bacterial disease is caused by organisms that are sensitive to standard antibiotics. Indeed the bug that causes one of the most feared infections – meningococcal disease – remains completely sensitive to penicillin.

The first thing I learnt when I started working with sexually transmitted infections (STIs) was that they aren't, well, sexy. Indeed, my initial decision to forge a career in STIs in the sphere of Aboriginal health would have been regarded by Sir Humphrey Appleby as courageous. Most doctors are reluctant to talk about sex and even my non-venereological infectious diseases colleagues are happy to leave STIs to the 'clap doctors'. Governments are not especially interested in STIs, even when one of them, chlamydia, has been the number one notifiable infectious disease in the country for over ten years. HIV may have changed things to some degree in the 1980s, but the other bugs received very little attention amid the millions of dollars of federal funding that went to HIV research and treatment. To redress this relative neglect, six chapters are devoted to STIs – a bias which I can further justify by observing that at least one in six readers of this book will acquire an STI in their lifetime – surely as good a motivation as any to read on!

Lastly, the book is a discontinuous narrative of some aspects of my medical life, but because each chapter is essentially self-contained the reader who likes to browse can dip into it at random. I have placed myself in most of the stories to give a first-hand perspective, but if the book appears to be a simple chronicle – or justification – of my career (such as it is), then I have failed in my intention.

1

Under the influence

Influenza A – an RNA virus that affects birds and mammals. Influenza A viruses are constantly changing. While humans who have been infected with one influenza strain in the past retain some degree of immunity to new strains, eventually a mutant appears that can overcome these defences and an influenza epidemic occurs. The word influenza is Italian for 'influence', and in medieval times the emergence of a flu epidemic was thought to be controlled by the stars – hence if someone was 'under the influence' it originally meant they had flu.

'I had a little bird/Its name was Enza/ I opened up the window/ And in-flu-enza… ' (children's skipping rhyme, c. 1918)

One of the great advantages of being a well paid specialist on the staff of a public hospital rather than a ridiculously well paid visiting medical officer in private practice is that you are entitled to long service and study leave. After ten years without a break of any substance, I was tired, grumpy, sick of being on call to the hospital, fed up with working on the weekend, short with my colleagues and occasionally dismissive of my students. I knew that soon I would reach that lowest of low points for a doctor – when you start to see patients as enemy; when you complain about them in the tea room as though they had contrived their illnesses just to annoy you. My family had started giving me concerned looks across the dinner table, and even my dog was keeping her distance.

So it was with considerable anticipation that I began a three-month sabbatical on 27 April, 2009. I was determined to make the leave count – I promised myself that I would be sitting at my desk every morning ready to write by no later than nine and, in an uncharacteristic display of planning, I had even constructed a timetable for the next 12 weeks. On the first morning, unshaved, wearing Ugg boots, tracksuit pants and tee-shirt, I drove my wife to work, returned home to read the paper slowly over breakfast, had a long shower – safe for once from spousal admonitions about water conservation – and arrived at my desk only a few minutes after my self-imposed deadline. I quickly scanned the top stories on the ABC News website and one item caught my eye.

'Experts say the swine flu outbreak currently stoking fears of a global epidemic poses a greater risk to Australia, with the onset of winter bringing the peak of the flu cycle.' I checked the BBC site: 'Schools in the capital city of Mexico are closed due to an outbreak of a disease called swine flu'.

Now this was strange – we had been expecting the next influenza pandemic to be caused by a mutation in the avian influenza virus, the H5N1 strain that mainly affected birds, not the H1N1 virus that was associated with pigs. I rang my wife, who works in infection control, and asked her what was going on.

'I can't talk, I have to go into a meeting with the chief health officer in a minute. There's a bit of a flap on in here.'

There were five infectious diseases specialists in our unit at the time. Two were on duty, one was overseas working on a project, one was in the Kimberley on holidays, out of phone range and I was … 'Oh no, you can't do this to me', I said out loud. I put down the phone and tried to concentrate on writing, without success. I turned on the radio and listened to the 10am bulletin. The top story was swine flu.

Influenza pandemics of the 20th century

There had been three influenza pandemics in the past 100 years – 1918, 1957 and 1968. The 1918 Spanish flu pandemic was the greatest natural disaster of the 20th century – estimates vary, but a minimum of 20 million and possibly up to 50 million people died, at least double the ten million who were killed on the battlefields of the First World War. In a world without antibiotics the secondary bacterial infections that followed the epidemic were often deadly, and there were no intensive care units (ICUs) to provide the care needed to allow patients time for their own immune system to win the fight against the pathogen. Around a third of the global population was infected with Spanish flu and more than 2.5 per cent of humanity died. The other pandemics were, by comparison, not in the same league: the Asian flu of 1957 is estimated to have caused around two million deaths worldwide, while the Hong Kong flu of 1968 is thought to have killed at most a million people.

I became intimately acquainted with Hong Kong flu as an eight year old; by nearly killing my father, the infection probably saved his life. I remember my father lying in the single bed in the spare room, the bedclothes pulled up over him as he shook his way through what I now know to be a rigour. When my mother had picked him up from the train station the previous night he had been completely well, but during the three-minute drive home he started complaining of chills and had started to shiver. By the time he had put his case down in the bedroom he could hardly talk because of the shaking. Hong Kong flu was on that evening's television news and on the front page of the day's *Sun*, so my mother had already made the diagnosis by the time our

GP arrived the next morning. He gave my father an injection in his bottom – everyone received penicillin in those days, even though doctors knew that antibiotics didn't work against viruses. I remember my mother's concern and the hushed kitchen conversations with friends who had never seen my father stopped by anything and suggested that he needed to go to hospital. He coughed and spluttered for weeks after the worst was over and he always remembered the illness as one of the worst he had experienced. He had smoked more than 20 cigarettes a day since the war, but after he recovered he never smoked again. He died at the age of 81.

Then for 40 years it was all quiet on the influenza front. There was a false alarm for a swine flu pandemic in 1975, but virologists believed that the next pandemic was not a matter of if but when.

Drift, shift, replication and re-assortment

There are three types of influenza virus – A, B and C. Pandemics are always caused by influenza A. Infection with influenza B can be severe but is rarely fatal and infection with C is uncommon and usually mild. The viruses have two main proteins on their surface – haemagglutinin (H) and neuraminidase (N) which are responsible for their confusing nomenclature. There are 16 N and 9 N subtypes but only H1, H2 and H3 and N1 and N2 commonly cause human disease. The Spanish flu and the 2009 swine flu were H1N1, the Asian flu was H2N2 and the Hong Kong flu was H3N2. Bird (avian) influenza is H5N1.

To understand why pandemics occur we need to understand a little about the way influenza viruses reproduce and how our immune systems respond to them.

Viruses commandeer the protein-making machinery of the body's cells to generate tens of thousands of copies of themselves. Every time a flu virus replicates (or copies) itself there is the potential for an error (mutation) to occur, resulting over time in significant changes to the structure of the virus and altering the way the host's immune system 'sees' it. After a first encounter with a virus it takes days or weeks for the immune system to produce specific antibodies against it, but if the same virus is encountered in the future the body's reaction time is much faster and the antibodies can destroy the virus before it has time to invade the human cell, replicate and cause disease. However, if a virus has mutated, the antibodies are unable to recognise it, giving the virus time to invade, replicate and cause disease all over again.

Some viruses mutate very little during replication. The measles virus that we are exposed to in childhood will be almost identical to the one that we may be re-exposed to decades later, and so immunity is life-long. The influenza A virus, however, is notable for its sloppy proof-reading and at least one mutation occurs with every copy. Most of these mutations are minor but when enough of them have accumulated by successive passages through infected human hosts, the structure of the virus at the end of the flu season may be quite different from the one at its beginning. This is known as antigenic drift, which, as the word 'drift' implies, is a gradual process which allows the human immune system to almost keep pace with viral evolution; you might be susceptible to next year's strain, but you are likely to have a least partial immunity. Antigenic drift won't lead to a pandemic – for that you need a sudden and profound change in the viral structure to produce a virus that no one in the population has previously encountered and developed immunity to – this seismic phenomenon is called antigenic *shift*. (It is important to point out that susceptibility is not the same as virulence: it is possible, as we will see, to have a pandemic that infects hundreds of millions but kills very few.) A shift requires more than just a few typos while transcribing the viral genetic code – it requires viruses to have sex with each other. Now, viral sex may be a difficult image to visualise (or not, I suppose, for many of the internet generation) but it really happens. Higher-order organisms such as us combine half their genetic material with half that of a member of the opposite sex to increase the genetic diversity of their offspring. Lower-order organisms mainly reproduce by making identical copies of themselves, but occasionally they display the more mature behaviour of their superiors. Sex between consenting viruses is more accurately, if less evocatively, known as re-assortment. A human influenza strain can re-assort with a bird or a pig strain and the resulting hybrid may have properties that produce very severe disease in humans. The frequently cited doomsday scenario is a re-assortment of the bird flu virus H5N1 with a human influenza virus that allowed bird flu to be transmitted from human to human. The reason infectious diseases specialists worry so much about such an event is that the world's insatiable appetite for poultry has produced a chicken population explosion, particularly in Asia. With so many birds living in close proximity to humans, viral re-assortments are occurring all the time and the emergence of a deadly strain is considered inevitable.

The 2009 swine flu pandemic

All epidemics start quietly – their early stages are usually undetectable by the routine surveillance mechanisms that health departments have in place. By the time you know that something is going on, the infectious agent is well established in the population. The swine flu virus responsible for the 2009 pandemic was first detected in Mexico in April, in four-year-old Edgar Hernandez who recovered completely, but the virus would have been circulating in the community for weeks or even months prior to this. Within a few days of Edgar's highly publicised diagnosis dozens of other people across Mexico were reporting fevers, muscle aches, and coughs. As I read the news bulletins each morning over the next few weeks it became clear to me that an antigenic shift had occurred. By the time the virus causing their symptoms was identified as swine flu (H1N1) in the Centers for Disease Control laboratory in Atlanta, Georgia, thousands more had been infected. The new virus was very similar in composition to the 1918 Spanish flu, but it was not clear if it possessed the same virulence as its 20th century ancestor. The World Health Organization (WHO) had been preparing for this event for more than a decade and an elaborate influenza pandemic plan had been formulated.

By the end of April 2009, cases of swine flu had been reported in the United States, Europe, India, Pakistan, Bangladesh and New Zealand. On June 11 Margaret Chan, Director-General of the WHO, told a press conference in Geneva: 'We are all in this together, and we will all get through this, together'. She had just declared the beginning of the first influenza pandemic of the 21st century.

Influenza is an autumn and winter disease, so though the virus was circulating in the northern hemisphere it was not expected to take off there until later in the year. The European and US public health communities were, therefore, closely watching the behaviour of the epidemic when it reached Australia and New Zealand during our winter. As had been predicted, attempts to contain the virus proved futile in a world interconnected by modern air travel, although many jurisdictions, including some in Australia, attempted to create a cordon sanitaire, reasoning that slowing the tempo of the epidemic even by a small degree would buy some time to get local plans in place.

One of the planks of the pandemic plan is the use of antiviral prophylaxis – the administration of a drug to people who are exposed to the virus to prevent them from contracting the illness and to break the chain of transmission. The antiviral agents that work against influenza – zanamavir (trade name Relenza – an Australian discovery) and oseltamivir (Tamiflu) – do not have anything approaching the potency that antibiotics have against severe bacterial infections. The anti-flu drugs inhibit the neuraminidase enzyme of the virus (the 'N' of H1N1) and as they have no effect on human cells they are very safe. The original studies that led to their licensing showed that patients with influenza who received either agent were, on average, free of symptoms for about one day less than those who received a placebo – a real but only modest benefit. Their effectiveness against serious, life-threatening influenza has never been subjected to a randomised clinical trial. Each country has established a national stockpile of the drugs, which are dispensed to those most in need during a pandemic – initially health care workers on the frontline of health care delivery. The problem with their use in prophylaxis is that they only work while you are taking them – if you stop the drug and are then re-exposed to influenza you can still become infected. Antiviral prophylaxis is a little akin to a First World War soldier donning a gas mask in the trenches when the mustard gas has been released – you are protected only as long as you have the mask on. To be able to safely discard the mask, to continue the metaphor, you need a ceasefire and this can only be achieved with vaccination.

Mild for most, fatal for a few

Influenza can manifest in many ways, from trivial and short-lived symptoms, such as a few muscle aches and a bit of a headache, to the disease that we all know as the flu – in which the symptoms range from severe muscle aches, feeling dreadful, high temperature, chills and uncontrollable shaking, through to life-threatening pneumonia, respiratory and other organ failure, and death. Every year thousands of people around the world die from what is known as seasonal influenza – but those affected are usually the frail and elderly members of the population and those with pre-existing serious chronic illness. During the 1918 pandemic the sequence of completely well, to moribund, to dead could occur within 24 hours and the disease targeted the younger and otherwise well members of the population.

We soon discovered that the 2009 swine flu was a mild disease in most people. There were exceptions: a fortnight after contracting swine flu two doctors at my hospital developed a neurological condition called Guillain-Barré, which damages the peripheral nerves and produces muscle weakness. One continued to work until he found himself unable to get out of the chair in his consulting room; the other woke to find himself unable to move the muscles of his face.

Our hospital was busy, but because the majority of those who were sick with the flu could be managed at home. There was no need for me to rush back to work and help my colleagues man the pumps. The smaller number of critically ill patients required the skills of the intensive care doctors, not my humble services. My wife gave me daily updates and, while subtly mentioning the important role she was playing, made it clear that I would just be in the way. At least my dog was talking to me again.

By July it was apparent that the death rate overall was between 0.001 and 0.03 per cent of those infected – much lower than the 0.1 per cent of the 1968 pandemic. The attack rate would turn out to be relatively low too – antibody testing performed after the epidemic ended would show that somewhere between 10 and 20 per cent of the population had been infected. But while some of us were busy reassuring the population that this was no 1918 Spanish flu, the intensive care doctors had witnessed something new and frightening: an epidemic of viral pneumonia that affected pregnant women, children and the middle-aged. In Australia, a total of 722 patients with H1N1 were admitted to an intensive care unit and 103 of these died, including seven pregnant women and seven children. Many more would have died if not for the heroic measures instituted in some cases – the sickest patients were treated with extra-corporeal membrane oxygenation (ECMO). This is the equivalent of putting someone on cardiac bypass for open-heart surgery, but instead of stopping after three hours you continue until the patient's lungs have recovered – which could take days or even weeks. ECMO is an expensive treatment that carries with it considerable risk of complications and can only be performed in a few specialist centres. After the epidemic was over, I attended a conference where the director of a major urban ICU said that during the epidemic his unit had reached the upper limit of its ability to cope with critically ill patients. If the number of cases had been any greater, he believed, the unit would not have been able to provide adequate care for all who needed it. In that event, many older people with complications of the flu who would otherwise have received intensive care would have been denied it to allow younger people, pregnant women and other high-risk patients access to treatment.

As it was, the absence of disease in the elderly was striking – the regular seasonal influenza targets mainly those over 65 – and was explained by data published in the *New England Journal of Medicine* showing that they had gained protection through exposure to a similar H1N1 strain in the past. All good doctors read the medical literature and learn from the published work of others, but the biased view that one gains from personal experience can be very difficult to shake. Many ICU doctors were perplexed and sometimes angered by the casual approach to the epidemic displayed by some of their non-ICU colleagues, who, lacking direct exposure to the sickest patients, and despite the published evidence, promulgated the belief that swine flu was no different from seasonal influenza.

Looking down the retrospectoscope

Criticism of the public health and medical response to the pandemic began to circulate almost as soon as the virus itself was identified. In Australia, the harshest comments were aimed at the vaccine policy. As we have seen, antigenic drift and shift allow flu viruses to evade the human immune system and new vaccines that anticipate these changes must be manufactured annually. There is no universal flu vaccine that will provide years of protection as there is with, say, polio, measles, and hepatitis B. Every year an expert WHO panel decides what antigens the new seasonal influenza vaccine should contain. (It is probably not too unfair to say that their deliberations are based on a mixture of experience, science and necromancy.)

The viruses chosen for inclusion must be inoculated into fertilised hens' eggs, and this is a laborious and complicated vaccine manufacturing process. New techniques for vaccine production are on the horizon, but the current methods are essentially the same as they were 50 years ago. In a pandemic setting, most manufacturers seek government underwriting as there are many commercial risks associated with the rapid roll-out of sufficient vaccine to cover an entire population. It takes four to five months to get a vaccine ready for distribution, by which time the epidemic may have already burnt itself out or been shown to cause only mild illness that wouldn't justify mass vaccination. Inevitably, there will be side-effects associated with the vaccine, and when tens of millions of doses are administered even vanishingly rare adverse reactions will occur, and indemnity against claims for harm may be required.

Within weeks of the beginning of the 2009 pandemic the Australian government contracted the pharmaceutical manufacturer CSL to produce 21 million doses of vaccine for the entire Australian population. The four-month lead time meant that the decision had to be made when the true virulence of the virus was not clear. It was not even known if one or two doses of vaccine would be required to produce adequate protection. To meet the unprecedented production demands, CSL had opted for multi-dose vials instead of the single-dose syringes that were usually supplied. The use of multi-dose vials has the potential for cross-contamination of blood-borne viruses and the decision was condemned by many infectious diseases experts *(see page 54)*. CSL argued that the risk of cross-infection was outweighed by the imperative of having enough vaccine ready in time. By the time it was available in September 2009 the low death rate had become apparent and the subsequent uptake of vaccine was modest, with less than a quarter of the population opting to receive it. Millions of doses were discarded.

The Australian federal government was loudly attacked in some medical quarters for wasting tens of millions dollars on the vaccine. State governments were criticised for their attempts at quarantine in the early weeks of the epidemic. The WHO was accused of having over-reacted by invoking its pandemic plan and of being conflicted because of the presence of pharmaceutical and vaccine producers on some of its expert panels.

There is a well known medical saying that things always look clearer through the retrospectoscope: what is self-evident in hindsight is hidden to us in prospect. While it is in its earliest stages it is impossible to predict the course of an epidemic with any degree of precision. The complexities of human behaviour, the unpredictability of the immunological response of the population and our rudimentary understanding of the basic biology of the influenza virus mean that an epidemic is only truly understandable *after* it has occurred. If the 2009 epidemic had turned out to have the same death rate as the Hong Kong flu we could have expected up to 4000 deaths; if it had mirrored the 1918 pandemic this number would have been ten or even 20 times higher. Arguments that modern care would prevent most of these deaths ignore the fact that the intensive care units were close to being overwhelmed by even the 'mild' 2009 virus.

Public health authorities have to follow the precautionary principle – they must exercise what is, in effect, a duty of care for the whole population. This means that even if there is only a small risk of something calamitous occurring we must prepare for it. The question is, of course, when does the risk become so small that we can ignore it. To act upon every risk would paralyse society, yet to ignore each could condemn it.

From where we stand now it is clear that the swine flu of 2009 was a novel and serious virus but not 'the big one'. Post-hoc analyses are essential in the public health outbreak domain and you have to own up to your mistakes if you have made any. Errors are inevitable in the face of uncertainty, and in the world of infectious diseases it is hard to think of anything as unpredictable as the behaviour of an influenza virus. Had the virus been more virulent and its death rate only twice as high as it actually was, those millions of dollars now seen as wasted on unused vaccine would have been just petty cash.

2

A beautiful anachronism

Penicillium notatum – a ubiquitous fungus that gets its name
from its resemblance under a microscope to a paintbrush (from
Latin penicillus: paintbrush). The fungus is harmless to humans
but one of the substances that it produces – penicillin – is toxic
to a wide variety of bacteria that can cause human disease.
Discovered by serendipity in 1928, its clinical potential was
overlooked until Howard Florey purified penicillin and began
animal experiments nearly a decade later.

'If penicillin can cure those that are ill, Spanish sherry can bring
the dead back to life.' (Sir Alexander Fleming, 1881–1955)

It was 1985 and we were sitting in the leather club chairs in the
doctors' lounge at Fairfield Infectious Diseases Hospital talking
about penicillin. Set in the urban bush, nestled beside the
Eastern Freeway that cleaves Melbourne in two, the hospital was
a beautiful anachronism. It was the last fever hospital operating
in Australia and in 11 years it would close forever. To step into
the grounds was to take a journey into the past, into a world
where people with infectious diseases were quarantined, brought
there by 'the black bus' that trawled the streets of the city picking
up contagious cases (and threatened to take my mother away
when she was a girl); a place of hushed corridors around the

tetanus patients; of the constant low-pitched whoosh, whoosh of the iron lungs in the polio wards. But it was the future too – here was the glorious over-reaction of the High Security Ward where haemorrhagic fever patients from Africa would go (if they ever came) and the high-technology laboratory where deadly viruses could be cultured. This was the world of novelist Michael Crichton's *The Andromeda Strain*: of doctors in space suits to protect them from alien airborne infections.

My affair with infectious diseases had begun in 1981, when I spent four weeks at Fairfield as a fifth-year medical student, and now, four years later, I was back and I was happy. A term at Fairfield was one of the most sought-after allocations at my 'home' hospital and to secure a junior resident position I had to effectively sacrifice the rest of my year in a round of bargaining with the medical administration.

The routine was to punctuate the morning ward round at 10.30 with a cup of tea and a discussion with the teams from the other wards. Each team consisted of a resident, registrar and one of Fairfield's consultant physicians. The consultants were permanent employees of the hospital, the registrars usually stayed for two years, and the residents rotated from a number of hospitals across the city. This was the last rotation of my second year after graduation, the end of my medical adolescence, and I would become a registrar in my next job.

It was September but still cold in the morning and a fire had been lit in the fireplace of the lounge. The windows looked out onto manicured gardens and you could watch the peacocks on the lawns strutting their stuff for the peahens. The sound of cars on the freeway was deadened by a dense ring of trees around the campus. The cafeteria adjacent to the lounge provided the best hospital food in Victoria, and you could even invite your girlfriend to dinner there and not be regarded as cheap. Only doctors were allowed in the lounge and my consultant, R., was already there, in his favourite chair, puffing on his pipe and filling the room with a fug of smoke. It is hard to believe now that he was allowed to smoke in the lounge, but at the time he was still railing against the not-so-distant prohibition of smoking in the wards themselves.

R. was the second most taciturn doctor I have met. He was grumpy and moody, but loved by most of the staff. He was the local expert on the clinical features of hepatitis, and had recently returned from a sabbatical in Atlanta, at the Centers for Disease Control, which was the epicentre for the study of the AIDS (acquired immune deficiency syndrome) epidemic. I had only been at the hospital for a few weeks and his quietness unnerved me a little. I would try to fill the silences with conversation, which mostly annoyed him.

'What was it like before penicillin?' I asked.

A smile formed on one side of his face. 'How old do you think I am?' he said.

After a quick calculation I realised that he must be in his mid-50s and he would have graduated when penicillin was at least 15 years old. He explained that he didn't know a medical world without antibiotics: we would have to consult *his* teachers to have a first-hand experience of the pre-antibiotic era.

Discoverer and developer

It was in 1928 that the British microbiologist Alexander Fleming discovered the antibacterial property of penicillin. He had prepared some agar plates that were growing the bacterium *Staphylococcus aureus* (see chapter 7) for an experiment, but had gone to France for the August holidays in the meantime. The plates were accidentally contaminated with a mould called *Penicillium notatum* and when Fleming returned he saw that the staph colonies had been inhibited in the areas where the mould was growing. He concluded that the mould was producing something that was killing the staph and called the substance peni-cillin. Fleming published his finding in 1929, but, lacking the biochemical expertise to isolate the compound, didn't pursue the research. In fact he doubted that penicillin would be of much use in combatting bacterial infections in humans, believing it would be inactivated too quickly.

It would be another ten years before the Australian-born pathologist Howard Florey would lead the research effort that demonstrated penicillin's value. With the biochemist Ernst Chain and others at Oxford, Florey developed a method of growing the mould and extracting enough penicillin to conduct experiments on mice. These were so conclusive that it was decided to treat a patient with an infection. The first person to receive intrave-nous penicillin was an Oxford policeman who had scratched his face on a rose thorn. He developed a serious spreading infection caused by a mixture of *S. aureus* and streptococci. By the time Florey saw him he was dying and had had one of his eyes removed. On 12 February 1941 the man received 200mg of penicillin (a tiny dose by today's standards). He responded dramatically to the first few infusions, but the penicillin soon ran out and he relapsed and succumbed to the infection. Later that year Florey and Chain carried their cultures across the Atlantic to the USA because there were no prospects of commercial production of the antibiotic in Britain. (Florey had secretly smeared the lining of his overcoat with *Penicillium* spores in case he was captured by the Germans on the way and his cultures were confiscated – though how he planned to recover the spores and recommence penicillin production in captivity was never explained.) Curing and preventing infections in the battle wounds of Allied troops in the latter part of the Second World War was hailed as one of miraculous uses of the new drug. Less well known is that peni-cillin revolutionised the treatment of gonorrhoea. Servicemen with gonorrhoea were considered unfit for active service, but the antibiotic returned thousands of men to active service – a mixed blessing indeed for those subsequently injured or killed on the battlefield.

The antibiotic era actually began in the mid-1930s, when a German scientist, Gerhard Domagk, showed that an aniline dye, sulphanilamide, had antibacterial activity. By 1939 sulphur drugs were widely available in medical practice and had been shown to reduce the death rate from puerperal fever – the streptococcal infection that can occur after childbirth *(see chapter 6)* – and to be effective in the treatment of meningitis and pneumonia. (Indeed it was a sulphur drug – sulphadiazine or 'M&B', after the makers May & Baker – that was used to treat the British war-time prime minister, Winston Churchill's, pneumonia in 1943.) Domagk was awarded the Nobel Prize for Medicine in 1939, but Hitler forbade him from accepting it because another recent German Nobel laureate had been openly anti-Nazi. It was sub-sequently awarded to him in 1947, two years after Florey, Chain and Fleming won their Nobel prize. This, plus the anti-German feeling of the post-war period, probably explains why penicillin was hailed as the first effective antimicrobial agent. (In fact, that distinction really belongs to Salvarsan, an arsenic-based com-pound used to treat syphillis, discovered by a Japanese scientist, Sahachiro Hata, in 1909 while he was working in the laboratory of the German giant of science, Paul Ehrlich.)

Keeping score

'The human race made it to 1945 without penicillin you know.' R. took another puff on his pipe and his face was obscured behind the smoke for a moment. 'The vast majority of people go through their life without needing antibiotics – really needing them, I mean.'

Before 1945 and the arrival of the widespread use of anti-biotics, humans had depended purely on the integrity of their immune system: the ability of the body to recognise harmful microscopic invaders and quickly mobilise components of the immune system to contain them, while also allowing the myriad of other organisms that cause no harm to happily coexist with us, which is one of the crowning achievements of evolution.

But what would happen to the patients with infections in hospital today if we didn't have any antibiotics? We thought about the patients we had seen that morning: a young man with an abscess in the muscles of his thigh that had required surgical drainage and which settled down quickly with intravenous antibiotics. It is axiomatic that pus must be surgically drained because antibiotics are unable to penetrate into an abscess and kill the bacteria contained within it, but the antibiotics reduce the effect that the infection has on the rest of the body: the temperature comes down, the patient feels better and the small number of organisms remaining are more easily mopped up by the immune system. So for that case we scored '1' for antibiotics, '1' for the immune system (and '1' for the surgeons). An elderly woman had been admitted the night before with pneumonia caused by a bacterium called *Streptococcus pneumoniae* (sometimes known as 'the old man's friend' in the pre-antibiotic era, so often did it provide a release from a lingering death for those who contracted it). The immune system ages along with the human it operates within – the old are more susceptible to infection because of a relative failure of their immunity, just as a newborn is at increased risk because of the system's immaturity. The woman was given intravenous penicillin and was looking much better that morning. We took the overall score to 2-1 for antibiotics. Then there was the 12-year-old girl who had been transferred from the country with symptoms consistent with meningitis. The cerebrospinal fluid that had been obtained from her lumbar puncture looked like pus and the same organism that we had identified in the old lady's blood – *S. pneumoniae* – had grown in the laboratory from this sample. (It was well known that bacterial meningitis was always fatal if untreated – contemporary audiences had been appalled by Harry Lime's dilution of the penicillin supplies for the children in the Viennese hospital in the 1949 film *The Third Man*.) This morning the girl was still sick but was expected to recover. We called this a clear victory to the antibiotics.

I suggested to R. that it must have been wonderful to have had a career that spanned the pre- and post-antibiotic eras. He was looking out the window at a peacock splaying its tail in front of one of the gardeners.

'I suppose it would have', he said.

Diagnosis: art or process

Doctors have to hold a lot of facts in their head, and the university selection process channels people into the profession with this basic but ultimately trivial skill. But as many a layperson knows if they have tried to work out what is wrong with them based on a comparison of their symptoms with what they have read in a textbook, it is really very difficult to make a diagnosis. Furthermore, treatment decisions seem simple in principle – diagnosis X gets drug Y – but it is another thing when you are actually faced with a sick person and they don't seem to be getting better after you have prescribed the appropriate therapy. This is when you need to measure yourself against a more experienced practitioner.

R's skill was in diagnosis. He always seemed to know what was going on with a patient. As junior doctors, we would see a patient, take the history, perform an examination and try to synthesise the information we had obtained to arrive at a sensible conclusion. This usually worked: we had enough experience to be able to match the data we had with a set of possible diagnoses. Sometimes, however, this process failed – the sum of the history, examination and investigations did not add up to a whole answer and we would be left with an unwell patient, without a clear idea of what was making them sick. When we presented the details of such a case to R. he would often offer a diagnosis that didn't make sense initially but ultimately proved to be the cause of the patient's illness. I remember one patient who had presented with weight loss and a fever that had been present for months. We had excluded the common things and the problem was now known as a PUO (pyrexia of unknown origin). In the days before there was a CT (computed tomography) scanner on every street corner, it was hard to exclude some particular diagnoses. R. listened to the history as I recounted it to him. 'He'll have a lymphoma', he said when I had finished. Some doctors have a constitutional feel for diagnosis – sometimes called heuristic understanding – but most don't. The ones who are good at it can't always explain how they came to a particular conclusion. Most doctors take a logical but slower path to diagnosis. (The patient was subsequently diagnosed with lymphoma.)

In the early 1980s R. had treated a group of homosexual men who had developed the symptoms of glandular fever but who tested negative for the agent that causes it – Epstein-Barr virus or EBV. The patients presented with fever and flu-like symptoms, sore throat and swollen lymph nodes in their neck and sometimes throughout their body. A rash was common. A diagnosis of sero-negative glandular fever had been made and the men's serum had been stored at the hospital. Fairfield had been collecting and freezing serum for nearly 40 years. Serum is the liquid part of blood that has had the red blood cells separated out by spinning at high speed in a centrifuge. The remaining clear yellowish liquid contains, among other things, antibodies produced by the immune system that can be tested many years after the sample is collected.

R. took me to see the serum banks that morning before our ward round. The specimens were kept in a row of rusting refrigerated shipping containers behind one of the wards. Inside them were rows of metal-topped small glass bottles, each with a label.

'I missed it, you know', R. said as we walked back to the common-room.

'There it was, right in front of all of us, and I missed it.' He sounded more rueful than distressed.

'Missed what?' I asked.

'They were all positive for HTLV-III', he replied. I asked him if he remembered the men's names.

'Not all of them – some. In fact, we're going to see a few of them on our ward round this morning', he said, tapping the ash from his pipe into the fireplace. We left the common-room and walked down the long, covered passage that led to Ward 4, and I began my first 25 years of working with the human immunode-ficiency virus.

3

Life during wartime

Human immunodeficiency virus – a member of the family
Retroviridae, HIV is an RNA virus that incorporates its own
genetic code into the DNA of the human cells that it infects.
CD4 lymphocytes, the white blood cells that make up the first
line of defence against retroviruses, carry a molecule that is
an exact fit for a protein on the surface of HIV. Like magnetic
limpet mines, the HIV particles attract the CD4 cells, bind to
them and initiate a permanent and incurable infection. Infected
CD4 cells slowly, but progressively, die off, making the infected
person vulnerable to one of the many infections and cancers
that constitute the syndrome known as AIDS.

'My thoughts are crowded with death/and it draws so oddly on
the sexual/that I am confused/confused to be attracted/by, in
effect, my own annihilation.' (from 'In Time of Plague', by Thom
Gunn, 1929–2004)

There were 16 patients with AIDS on Ward 4. They were all men,
all homosexual, and they were all dying.

In 1985 it felt as though the clocks had turned back to a
time before penicillin. Before the emergence of HIV, there was
a pervading belief that the age of description and discovery in
microbiology was over: the Australian Nobel laureate Macfarlane

Burnet signalled 'the end of infectious diseases' in a number of his lectures and books in the 1970s. Smallpox was gone, polio was going, and pneumonia didn't kill young people any more. Rheumatic fever was a rarity – among white Australians anyway – and it was now time to hand the research baton to those investigating cancer, a disease that predominantly affected the ageing population. So the appearance of a virus that seemed to slowly kill everyone who contracted it was as much a shock for the medical world as it was for the general population. Just four years previously reports had started to emerge from San Francisco and New York of clusters of gay men with strange infections that were usually only seen in people being treated for cancer, and of an increase in cases of a rare tumour called Kaposi's sarcoma. Cases among injecting drug users, both straight and gay, and in heterosexuals from Haiti were also appearing. Initially the cause was suspected to be related to lifestyle factors, such as using the recreational 'popper' drug amyl nitrate, but when patients whose only risk factor was being the recipient of a blood transfusion started to be diagnosed it was clear that the illness was caused by a transmissible agent.

Within just three years of the first appearance of the illness that was originally known as gay-related immune deficiency (GRID), the virus that caused AIDS was discovered by the then unknown French virologists Luc Montagnier and Françoise Barré-Sinoussi. They called the virus LAV, short for lymphadenopathy-associated virus. The Americans were close behind and called their virus HTLV-III (human T cell lymphotropic virus III). Robert Gallo, the US researcher whose earlier work on retroviruses had paved the way for the discovery by the French team, claimed precedence for the discovery of the AIDS virus. A bitter, decade-long dispute ensued, finally resulting in a truce whereby joint discovery was acknowledged. However, Gallo was not included in the 2008 Nobel Prize for Medicine, which was awarded to Montagnier and Barré-Sinoussi.

In 1986 it was agreed that the virus belonged in a class of its own and it received its official and permanent title – human immunodeficiency virus or HIV. The worst epidemic of the 20th century was caused by a virus of unprecedented indolence, one that could be transmitted through private and pleasurable activity and from people who didn't know that they were sick.

Dozens of AIDS-defining illnesses were being identified and everyone was learning about their clinical manifestations and treatment on the run– there was no textbook to read, no store of collected wisdom among clinicians. It was a great leveller – a young doctor could contribute to new knowledge as much as an experienced clinician. For example, my first academic paper, on the treatment of PCP (pneumocystis carinii, now jiroveci, pneumonia) – the most common opportunistic infection in people with HIV at the time (see chapter 4) – was published in The Lancet when I was in my second year after graduation. I had no idea then how hard it was to get something accepted by The Lancet, but the international attention that AIDS was receiving smoothed the path of my paper to publication.

We soon discovered, to our horror, that a patient who was diagnosed with what we then called full-blown AIDS had a 50 per cent chance of being dead within 12 months, and close to 100 per cent of those so diagnosed were dead within two years.

HIV specifically targets one class of white blood cells: the CD4 (or helper T4) lymphocyte. The CD4 cell has a number of receptor molecules on its surface, one of which is a perfect fit for a protein on the outer surface of the HIV virus called gp120. This has to be one of the best 'tricks' in infectious diseases – here is a virus that appears to be designed to neutralise the very cell that under normal circumstances would be responsible for destroying it. No wonder, perhaps, that early in the epidemic conspiracy theories circulated that the virus had escaped from a US military laboratory where it had been created as a biological warfare agent.

The CD4 cell has a co-ordinating role in the body's immune response to infection and stands at the centre of one of the most complex processes in biology. It has been described as the conductor of the immune orchestra: in the absence of a full complement of CD4 cells, all the distinct components of the immune system can still play their individual tune but they do not know how to stay in touch with the other members. Some play *allegro* when they should be *lento*; others *piano* when they should be *forte*. The isolated depletion of CD4 cells, and the patterns of illness that occurred as a result, had never been seen before.

Infection with HIV soon impairs the function of the CD4 cells. Over several years their absolute number declines. On average, between six and eight years after infection, the number of CD4 cells falls to a critical level and the patient's immune system is unable to control infections that, in the normal host, would be easily dealt with.

The end result of the CD4 shortage is immunosuppression – the commonest causes of which among Australians include the drugs used to suppress the immune system in patients with kidney and heart transplants, the chemotherapy given to cancer patients, and, increasingly, the drugs used against chronic diseases such as rheumatoid arthritis and inflammatory bowel disease. Such immunosuppression is described as iatrogenic (brought on by treatment – from the Greek 'iatros', meaning 'physician'). The type of infections that immunosuppressed people are at risk of depends on the specific impairment in the immune system caused by their treatment and on the range of pathogens that they have been exposed to in their lifetime.

The commonest AIDS-defining illnesses are the aptly named opportunistic infections. The germs that cause these illnesses are usually of such low virulence that they are kept in check by a normal immune system: they only manifest as disease when the patient's immunity is profoundly compromised. For example, most women will have been troubled by vaginal thrush at some time in their life and considered it to be a temporary nuisance. For the HIV-infected patient, however, the fungus that causes thrush – *Candida albicans* – can infect the entire length of the oesophagus, causing excruciating pain and impairing the ability to eat. A viral infection called cytomegalovirus or CMV, to which over 80 per cent of the population have been exposed by the time they reach adulthood but which rarely causes problems, can infect the retina of the HIV patient and rapidly lead to blindness. A fungus that is only rarely found in the general population – *Cryptococcus neoformans* – causes life-threatening meningitis in at least 10 per cent of AIDS patients.

Even after just a few years of infection, while maintaining normal levels of CD4 cells, patients with HIV have a much greater risk of being infected by pathogens – the most important of which is *Mycobacterium tuberculosis*, the cause of TB. Although not a major problem in the developed world, nearly a third of the population living in the developing world have been exposed to TB and carry a small number of the organisms in their body. This latent infection can re-activate in an otherwise healthy person, but it occurs at a much higher rate among people infected with HIV.

It is not only infections that are amplified by HIV. The immune system is also important in the control of cancers. A rare tumour called Kaposi's sarcoma, which was thought to affect only elderly Ashkenazy Jews, is common in late HIV infection. Lymphoma (cancer of the lymph glands) is also a frequently encountered HIV-related neoplasm.

The testing and counselling quandary

The first antibody tests for AIDS became available in 1985. While they picked up almost everyone with the disease, the tests were not very specific, meaning a lot of people without HIV infection tested positive. No test performs perfectly, but one that told you incorrectly that you had a disease that appeared to be inevitably fatal had the potential to cause considerable harm. Australia was one of the first countries to secure its blood supply through testing of donations, but in the process hundreds of false-positive test results were returned, alarming the donors who had to suffer through months of anguish before they were found to be clear of infection.

The thousands of homosexually-active men who knew that they could have contracted HIV in the preceding four or five years faced a difficult decision. Everyone in the gay community knew someone who had developed an illness consistent with AIDS, but it was plain that there was a long gap between the time of infection and the development of conditions indicative of AIDS. There was heated and, at times, acrimonious debate in the community and among the medical profession about the utility of HIV testing. Even if we assumed that the early antibody tests performed perfectly – which they certainly didn't – would you want to know that you were HIV positive? During the years that it took for the virus to deplete the immune system most people felt well and showed little or no sign of the infection. If you were a gay man and knew that you were at risk of infection but you felt well, why would you give yourself a sudden and irreversible indication that you were going to die sooner rather than later? At the time there was no treatment that would reverse the immunosuppression, so early diagnosis was of limited benefit to the patient. If you were HIV positive you would not be able to get life insurance, and in the case of doctors it could exclude you from working in some specialty areas, such as surgery.

Those on the other side of the argument reasoned that by knowing you were HIV positive you could prevent transmission to others by practising safe sex – using condoms with every sexual act. But this knowledge was redundant if you always practiced safe sex regardless of your HIV status. There *was* some medical benefit in knowing you had the disease – the use of anti-biotics and antifungals could delay the onset of AIDS by a few years, and the early identification of AIDS-related infections was associated with a higher rate of survival than if the diagnosis was made when the patient was very sick. While community groups tended to argue against testing for people without symptoms, there were advocates of both positions among the medical profession and some in the community. Because of this uncertainty the concept of pre-test and post-test counselling was developed – one that still exists 20 years later and which has been both a boon and a burden.

Pre-test counselling was designed to ensure that anyone who was tested for HIV was made aware of the significance of a positive result and the possible implications. It also explained how a negative result may not be correct because you might be in the 'window period' – that time when the virus is circulating in the blood but the immune system hasn't yet made antibodies against it. Conversely, a positive test might not represent a true infection. Pre-test counselling was also an opportunity to reinforce the need for safe sex and safe injecting. The new process for testing for HIV was a major change in medical practice. Previously, few doctors had seen the need to seek informed consent for a simple blood test, but with the advent of HIV the community and the profession realised what the implications of this elementary procedure could be. There was a spill-over effect into other areas of medicine too: it was realised that consent was required for other diagnostic procedures, such as genetic testing.

Unfortunately, the requirement for pre- and post-test counselling also created the widespread belief that testing for HIV could only be done by designated pre-test counsellors and that the process required at least an hour, sometimes longer. These misconceptions still persist in many quarters today, even though medical students are taught otherwise. The culture of the 'real' medical world is such that some new graduates think that there is something special about HIV testing. The perceived need to talk about sex and illicit drugs puts many general practitioners off and deters them from testing. The fact that many doctors are unintentionally discouraged from HIV testing has probably resulted in little harm in Australia because HIV remains an uncommon infection among people outside the at-risk groups. But some harm is done; Elizabeth McDonald, when working with me as a medical student, showed that, apart from 'gay-identifying' men, every patient who was diagnosed with HIV in the Australian Capital Territory in a ten-year period had been seen by a doctor at least once, and usually several times, before an HIV diagnosis was finally made. (I am often bemused when a patient is referred to me with a complex problem and I find they have had every test under the sun performed – except for HIV. The hepatitis B and C test has been done, but the referring doctor has stopped short of an HIV test because, I have learnt, they felt that they weren't able to do the pre-test counselling.)

In 2006 I chaired the committee that revised the Australian HIV testing guidelines. We re-emphasised that pre-test counselling should be termed pre-test information to make it easier for non-specialists to order HIV testing. We also recommended that all pregnant women should be offered an HIV test, something which had been a contentious issue for 20 years. Community groups had been worried that HIV-positive women would be tested without their consent, while many HIV specialists argued that identification of HIV during pregnancy would allow treatment of the mother, which almost completely eliminates the risk of transmission to the unborn child. This is a very real issue for me: I have many female patients with HIV, some of whom have children who are also infected with HIV. The women who were found to be HIV positive in early pregnancy received antiviral treatment and none of their children are infected. Unfortunately these guidelines, like many, have had little effect on the average doctor's practice.

In sub-populations at higher risk and in countries with a larger proportion of HIV infections testing is a major component of public health strategy, and in these settings it is crucial to get the balance right between informed consent and real-world practise.

From illicit thrill to sombre reflection

My rotation as a resident at Fairfield lasted only three months before I had to leave to commence my physician training elsewhere. When I left we all knew that AIDS was a terrible disease, but some of us, perhaps all of us, were quietly excited. By the time I returned three years later as a senior registrar, however, the staff had watched a cohort of young men prematurely age and die in front of them, and the illicit thrill of working with a new disease had given way to something more sombre, more respectful.

I saw bodies that were held together by just skin and sinew, the fat and muscle having dissolved as the disease progressed. Some patients became my friends and then died. Some friends became my patients and they died too. This wasn't supposed to happen: I had become accustomed to looking after old people who were dying. Young people had, of course, died before the advent of HIV, but such deaths were punctuations of sadness, intermittent tragedies. At Fairfield, I witnessed a relentless march of physical corruption that was killing people out of time, like a latter-day bubonic plague. Gay men sat with their dying lovers or good mates, who cleaned up their shit and piss, wiped the sweat from their foreheads and backs, changed the vomit-covered sheets, and smelt the decay rising up from inside once beautiful bodies. And every day they had to hide the awful truth from themselves – that this was the future for many of them too. This modern prophecy was fulfilled in slow motion. It was not possible to know when you would die – perhaps next year, perhaps in a more distant future –only that it would be sometime too soon. I couldn't understand how they coped with this realisation. Some did sink into despair, others into a manic hedonism, but the love that these men had for each other kept them afloat and laughing. The dying wards were full of life and music. Cups of sorrow were often filled with tears of joy.

I watched mothers grieving for their dying sons – mothers who supported one another, while the fathers sat quietly alone in the corner of the room and tried to say the things that they knew they should, and fought to keep to themselves the things they knew they shouldn't.

The suffering of death was apparent to us every day: the pain of the Kaposi's sarcoma tumours that compressed nerves and made faces swell into grotesque masks, and caused bodies to bloat and ulcerate. I am not an animal, I am … what am I? I am dying. Handsome men became hideous to themselves, and we sometimes covered the mirrors in their rooms. We had no idea how many people were going to be infected – the threat to the entire population was real, and some people who today say that there was never really anything to worry about were at the time speaking in apocalyptic terms.

The corruption of certainty

Life during wartime. The Talking Heads song kept playing in my head: 'This ain't no party, this ain't no disco, this ain't no foolin' around'. I had read Susan Sontag at university and knew her cautions against military metaphors but I couldn't help drawing parallels. Everything changes in war – standard operating procedure is suspended, certainties become relativities, absolute truth dissolves in absolute alcohol. Living for a moment in the penumbra of death intensifies the glare of life – and, over time, black and white morality began to fade to shades of grey.

We started to hear stories of people outside of the hospital who were being gently helped across the line into the long dreamless sleep of death. What was shocking about providing a guarantee that relief would come quickly and certainly? How could this not be right? How could we ignore the suffering, we were asked. How could we refuse to provide the drugs.

Many of the staff were gay and their close connection with the community made the daily work of caring even more poignant. Some staff were infected and the knowledge provided them with nothing but fear. And those of us who were straight and uninfected knew that there was only a needlestick between us and them: the price of freedom, eternal vigilance.

And then signs began to appear that the worst was over: not an unconditional surrender but a negotiated truce. By 1990 the number of new cases of infection in Australia was falling. Safesex education was funded and promoted by a commonwealth government and parliament possessed of an unprecedented – and probably never to be repeated – wisdom in the sphere of public health. Due to the introduction of needle and syringe exchange programs the infection rate among injecting drug users, who were believed to be the bridge between the gay and straight populations, remained less than 1 per cent. A new cohort of young, uninfected gay men moved onto the scene. To protect themselves from infection they warned each other not to have sex with old men – and I realised that they meant as old as me.

My generation's penicillin

In 1992 I moved to the Northern Territory. One of my motivations for leaving Melbourne was a desire to dilute my medical practice with more living than dying patients. Nevertheless, I had about 50 HIV-infected patients who attended my clinic

in Darwin and, although treatment was improving incremen-
tally, most of them were slowly deteriorating. I cared for many
patients in their last months and weeks.

But in June 1996 something incredible happened. Just 12
years after HIV had been identified, highly active antiretroviral
therapy became available – a cocktail of drugs that gave the rather
touching acronym HAART. The results from clinical trials had
shown that the effect was stunning – complete suppression of
the virus could be achieved even in patients with advanced HIV
infection (those with a very low CD4 cell count). As a result, I
watched my patients' CD4 counts start to rise out of the danger
zone and, in some cases, into the normal range. It was too early
to be certain – the sustainability of the response to treatment
could not be known at that time – but it was clear that we were
on the verge of something very exciting. In fact, we were wit-
nessing one of the extraordinary medical advances of the 20th
century. This was my generation's penicillin. I would talk to my
own residents in years to come of the days before HAART and
those after HAART. Combination therapy could not have come
at a better time – the HIV epidemic, while essentially static in
Australia, was accelerating elsewhere. Sub-Saharan Africa, India,
and parts of southeast Asia had seen an explosion of cases, and
by the 1990s up to a third of the sexually active population in
some African countries was infected.

On 1 July that year the world's first euthanasia legislation
(*The Rights of the Terminally Ill Act*) came into operation in the
Northern Territory. It had been passed the previous year but it
had taken 12 months to finalise the regulations that would guide
its implementation. I had publicly opposed the legislation. The
euthanasia debate was carried out in a region that was in the
middle of an epidemic of suicide in young Aboriginal people
in remote communities (that continues to this day) and where
Aboriginal adults died 20 years earlier than their non-Aboriginal
friends and neighbours. I found it hard to contain my irritation:

how could this be a priority? Why would you choose this particular social reform when there were so many more that could improve the lives of people in the Territory? The time we spent worrying about the euthanasia bill was time not available for the daily, pressing needs of the Aboriginal population. Indeed, some of us believed that the Bill was more than just a distraction: that it was actually a threat to Aboriginal people. Trust between Aboriginals and the health services was always fragile, and there were reports that bush people were frightened to come into town because they believed that the whitefellas were killing their sick people. Delay in presentation to medical services was already an important problem and here was another reason to stay away from the clinic.

I could support the deliberate hastening of the death of a patient when physical suffering was extreme and unbearable, where there was no further treatment available, when there was no hope of recovery and death was imminent. Every doctor and nurse with clinical experience will have cared for patients who meet these criteria and many would be willing to hasten and even cause death when faced with such a clinical circumstance. But the Northern Territory legislation was not just concerned with the very end of life – the regulations were worded in such a way that a person who had received a diagnosis of terminal illness could legally seek euthanasia at the moment of diagnosis if, in the opinion of their doctor and a specialist in the illness in question, they had less than a year to live. The wise doctor knows that it is impossible to tell a patient exactly how long they have to live – studies can tell us what the average survival time is for patients of the same gender, and similar age and disease states, but only a foolish doctor gives a specific time. If they do, it is almost always wrong: patients who look like they will live for six months are sometimes dead in two, and others who you expect to die in a few months are still alive two years later. It is one thing to assist the death of a patient who is clearly in a terminal phase but another to assist one who, apart from having been given a dreadful diagnosis, appears well and full of life.

As the legislation stood, almost every one of my HIV-positive patients could theoretically have met the criteria for euthanasia – they all had an incurable illness which *could* kill them within 12 months, although only those whose immune systems were profoundly impaired would have been likely to die in the next year. But the death rate of patients with HIV with only mild immunosuppression was many times higher than that of their non-infected counterparts and I have no doubt that it would have been possible to make an argument for euthanasia for them too. A few weeks later I received a letter from a man in Melbourne with AIDS. He had been at my school and, although we were not close friends, our orbits had occasionally intersected. He had contracted HIV in the 1980s and now he was in the late stages of the disease. He had developed CMV retinitis and was going blind. At that time CMV infection was a harbinger of death – the average time left for someone who was diagnosed with it was about eight weeks. He asked if I would look after him if he moved to the Territory.

'I want you to do euthanasia on me', he wrote.

I had cared for many AIDS patients at his stage of the disease, so I was aware how sick he would be. Moving to the tropics when you are fit and well is hard enough because of the extreme humidity and heat, but it would be a nightmare for someone in his state. I know that there were hundreds of people like my old school acquaintance who would have been tempted to avail themselves of the euthanasia legislation prior to the advent of the new drugs. I also know that most of them are still alive today. I don't want to overstate the potential for the emergence of new treatments as an argument against euthanasia, because the discovery of HAART was a once in a medical lifetime breakthrough. There is, arguably, no other condition except AIDS for which the prognosis has changed so dramatically in the past 20 years.

I could not have had the same sense of optimism for patients with pancreatic cancer or advanced liver cancer, where the gains in survival have been very modest. But the suffering of young patients with advanced HIV infection had been part of the community's emotional priming for the euthanasia campaign, and now, unexpectedly, it was in this specific area that the need for the legislation was suddenly diminished and its inherent weaknesses exposed.

I wrote back to my friend that I would be pleased to see him, that I would treat him with the antiviral drug that could delay the progression of CMV retinitis and I would apply to the federal government to get him onto the recently released combination of HIV medications. I could not in conscience perform euthanasia on him, I explained, but would do all in my power to help him if he did not respond to the anti-HIV medication. I sent the letter with a heavy heart but I never received a reply. I hope against hope that he is still alive.

4

The pricking of my thumb

Pneumocystis jirovecii – a yeast-like fungus often found
in normal lungs but which can cause a severe pneumonia
in patients with depressed immunity. The first epidemic
of pneumocystis pneumonia (PCP) was recorded in
malnourished children after the Second World War, but in
the 1980s it became the commonest infection associated
with AIDS. The symptoms of PCP are mild to begin with
and can take several weeks to reach a point where the
immunosuppressed patient seeks medical attention. If
untreated it is invariably fatal.

'By the pricking of my thumbs, something wicked this way
comes … ' (from *Macbeth*, by William Shakespeare, 1564–1616)

During the last week of September 1989 I admitted a seriously
ill man to Fairfield. The patient – I'll call him Peter J – was in his
40s. In the preceding few weeks he had noticed that he couldn't
swim his usual number of laps in the pool and over the previous few days he had struggled to even climb the stairs to his
second-floor flat. He had woken several times in the past week
with drenching sweats and had to change his nightshirt. By the
time he saw his GP Peter J was breathless after the most trivial
exertion and had struggled to make it to the surgery. Although

he had never been tested for HIV before being admitted to Fairfield, he had his suspicions: this was the decade when every gay
man had a friend or lover dead or dying of AIDS.

The GP referred his patient to us, and as Fairfield didn't have
an emergency department, he was transferred immediately to
Ward 4. A chest X-Ray had shown the ground-glass haziness in
both his lungs that is characteristic of a condition called pneumocystis pneumonia (PCP).

The organism that causes PCP, *Pneumocystis jirovecii*, can be
found in the lungs of most healthy people, where it sits quietly
and causes no problems. It had been first identified in the laboratory early in the 20th century and was classified as a protozoan –
in the same kingdom as malaria. The first human cases were not
diagnosed until after the Second World War, but by the 1970s it
was known to be a rare complication of the immunosuppression
associated with cancer treatments and the anti-rejection drugs
given to patients with organ transplants. One of the first clinical
clues to the emergence of the HIV epidemic in the early 1980s
was the sudden increase in requests to the Centers for Disease
Control in Atlanta from doctors in New York and San Francisco
for permission to use one of the restricted drugs effective against
PCP. Soon PCP was the most common AIDS-defining condition
and we became quite skilled in diagnosing and treating it. (In
the last decade analysis of the organism's DNA has shown it to
be a fungus not a protozoan – a somewhat surprising finding
considering that the drugs used to treat it have no effect on any
other fungi.)

Blood taken from the radial artery of Peter J's wrist – a test
far more painful and more difficult to perform than the usual
blood sample, which is drawn from a vein on the inside of the
elbow – revealed that his oxygen level was dangerously low. We
moved him to the Intensive Care Unit at the other end of the
hospital, where, despite high doses of antibiotics, he continued
to deteriorate over the next 24 hours until he reached a point

where he had to be sedated and intubated to maintain an adequate level of oxygen in his blood.

I was covering the ICU that evening and received a phone call from the nursing staff saying that the patient had suddenly deteriorated. His blood pressure had fallen, his pulse was 140 – nearly twice normal – and his oxygen level was just holding at a point consistent with life. Unlike the bigger Melbourne ICUs, which looked after complicated trauma, post-surgical and cardiac patients, this was a small unit that, perhaps unique among such places, had an almost homely feel to it. It was not unusual to be startled during a ward round by the appearance of one of the resident peacocks that had flown onto the roof and was squawking through the skylight windows. While the four or five patients in the ward were dependent on the life-support machines for their survival, the sense of controlled drama that the bigger units almost revelled in was missing here. Fairfield's experience in nursing the remaining survivors of the last Australian polio epidemics had made the staff expert at caring for patients who needed to rely on a ventilator for months or even years. None of our staff specialists had been specifically trained in ICU and we relied upon the experience of the older consultants who had grown up in a time when they had to do everything themselves – intubation, tracheostomies (where a breathing tube is inserted into the lungs via an incision made in the trachea below the thyroid gland in the neck), dialysis, and so on. Although it would be hard to argue that the younger consultants were at the cutting edge of advances in the management of critically ill patients, they were fine and committed physicians and had no hesitation trying to prolong the life of their young, doomed HIV patients, who might have been refused intensive care treatment in the other hospitals.

(This was a transition period for Fairfield: an independent review by two interstate infectious diseases specialists had recently recommended that the personnel and patients be moved to another Victorian tertiary hospital where the facilities to perform complicated, but increasingly routine, radiological investigations were available and where there was better surgical support. We didn't, for example, have a CT scanner, and although we had an operating theatre there was no resident anaesthetist or surgeon. The staff had rejected the findings of the review and had begun fighting the state government, which had signalled its intent to close the hospital. I got caught up in the fight and fiercely defended the hospital's right to stay open. Later I changed my view, which led to some senior staff seeing me as 'one of them'.)

I walked into the ICU with the sense of heightened awareness that you need to possess in these circumstances. You know that you are being summonsed to attend a minor crisis but don't have the information necessary to determine its cause as you enter the room. You have to listen to the staff who are briefing you as well as take in the visual clues. You have to *look* cool as well as *be* cool while you digest the facts and come to a conclusion. I had been called to a patient with a similar problem earlier in the year and had missed the correct diagnosis, so I was determined not to make the same mistake again.

'I was just changing the dressing on his drip when his BP [blood pressure] dropped and his sats [blood oxygen saturation level] fell', the nurse told me.

I put my stethoscope on the front of the patient's chest. I couldn't hear the normal sounds of air moving in the left lung and there was a slight deviation of his trachea to the right – this latter sign was subtle and I wasn't convinced that it was true or if I was just making it up to fit in with the diagnosis that was firming in my mind, which was that Peter J had developed a pneumothorax, a well recognised complication of PCP, especially when the patient is intubated. The increased pressure flow through the tube inserted down the throat can blow a hole in one of the lungs and air leaks out into the space between the lung and chest cavity. The lung collapses as a result and the patient is then firing on one cylinder. In the typical out-of-hospital setting, a spontaneous pneumothorax occurs in fit, tall, young males and the consequences are serious but rarely life-threatening. When the patient is already sick and their oxygenation level is low, it can be a fatal complication, especially if a tension pneumothorax occurs. If this complication was present, the pressure outside the lung would be increasing with each additional inspiration and the heart would be being pushed to one side of the chest, eventually impeding its ability to pump. It was after-hours, when normally the radiographer would have left, but luckily he was still in the hospital car park when he was paged (mobile phones were only 'car phones' in those days and were the preserve of rich doctors). In the meantime I had to decide if we needed to urgently drain the air from the chest with a needle inserted between the ribs.

I stood back from the bed and took a few quiet breaths myself – in an emergency always take your own pulse first – and I looked again at the monitors and back to the patient. His blood pressure was holding up, just, and the measure of oxygen in his blood was borderline. I decided to wait until the X-ray was taken unless these parameters changed in the next few minutes. We had the portable X-ray back in ten minutes and it confirmed the presence of a pneumothorax, but there was no evidence of any displacement of the heart – apparently all the tension was in me, not the patient. This finding meant that I could drain the air from his chest in a slightly more leisurely fashion. The nurse had set up a tray for the sterile pack which contained the necessary items for the insertion of an intercostal tube. The principle is straightforward – make a small hole in the chest and stick in a tube to drain the air out. But even the simplest medical procedure can go very wrong if not performed properly. After I applied an antiseptic solution to the skin on the side of his chest about 15 cm below the armpit, I injected local anaesthetic into the skin and deeper tissues. I then made an incision with a scalpel, first through the skin and then deeper into the muscle between the fifth and sixth ribs. I opened up the track made by the incision with forceps until their tip was within the chest cavity – there was a faint rush of escaping air – and then I inserted the plastic intercostal tube into the chest. There was a clamp at the end of the tube, which I released once it was connected to a bottle half-filled with water, which creates a one-way valve system that allows air to escape from the chest through the tube but none to enter the tube, and the patient, from the outside. The vigorous bubbling of the underwater drain confirmed that the system was working, and within a few minutes the patient's blood pressure rose and his oxygen saturation had returned to normal.

I found the performance of this kind of procedure one of the most satisfying parts of my job as I felt that I had really done something for my patient. The prolonged 'childhood' of medical school and the 'teenage years' of junior doctoring can be frustrating, but in this case I had made a diagnosis and then instituted a course of action that had fixed the problem. If you do the procedure properly – dexterously and quickly – you also receive tacit praise from the nursing staff, who, after years of assisting in such situations, know who is good and who isn't. I had done dozens of intercostal tubes during my training and I could sense the approval of the nurse who was helping. It was with a feeling of some pride, therefore, that I finished the job by fashioning an elegant roman-sandal suture that was then the accepted way of fastening the tube to the chest wall to stop it from falling out.

With what should have been the last pass of the suture needle through the skin I encountered more resistance than I anticipated. I was using my other hand to stabilise the skin around the tip of the soon to re-emerge suture when the resistance suddenly gave way and the needle shot out of the skin, through my glove and into my thumb. I didn't say anything and hoped that the nurse hadn't seen it happen. It looked clumsy and, I know this sounds hard to believe, I was at that moment more concerned about looking competent in the eyes of the staff than worrying about the fact that I had just stuck myself with a needle that had been pushed through the skin and muscle of a patient in the late stages of HIV infection. I carried on as though nothing had happened to me, applied the dressing and checked that the tube was still draining properly. It was only when I was sure that everything was in order that I took off the two pairs of surgical gloves that I was wearing and examined my thumb. There was no sign of blood. I checked the gloves – no tell-tale stain there either. I could see a little scratch on the surface of my skin, but the needle had hardly breached the epidermis, the most superficial layer.

My next step should have been to notify one of the other doctors that I had suffered a needlestick injury. The new drug AZT (zidovudine), had recently become available in Australia and there was already some evidence that it reduced the risk of transmission of HIV following a needlestick injury. I cannot really explain why I didn't tell anyone about the injury or think about taking AZT prophylactically. Perhaps I thought that the scratch was only trivial and the risk of transmission was small: the needle was for suturing, so not a hollow-bore type, and it had passed through two layers of latex glove before it glanced my skin. Regardless of what I thought, I was breaking a hospital rule – if it was known that a nurse had been involved, an incident report would have been filled in and a clear process followed. Doctors are notorious for not reporting incidents like this and I knew that several of my registrar colleagues and consultant bosses had had unreported exposures. (The following year I wrote a paper on needlesticks based on the information systematically collected at Fairfield over the preceding six years, so by then I knew the procedure well. There is a pop-psychology explanation for my unconscious motivation in writing the article, which strongly argued for a coherent follow-up process in the event of an occupational exposure to HIV.)

I left the patient in the ICU and went home after my shift ended to contemplate the next three months – the time I would have to wait until I knew that I had not been infected. I was married and we had a newborn baby at home. The fact that I have no recollection of who was playing or won the next day's AFL grand final reveals, at least for Victorian readers, how occupied my thoughts were with the incident and its possible repercussions. I looked at my thumb the next morning – there was no evidence of any mark forming to reveal the originally invisible scratch. I continued to rationalise the low infection risk throughout the weekend and on returning to work on the Monday morning wrote 'HIV test' in my pocket diary on a page 90 days in the future. I tried to do my ward round as though nothing had happened.

In a climate of fear

It was understandable that a disease like HIV would cause panic in the general population when it first appeared, but it was unforgivable that some members of the medical profession mirrored and in some cases amplified the fear. Although my time at Fairfield as a junior resident had metaphorically immunised me against AIDS hysteria, the fact that the hospital itself was isolated from the rest of the city and that its looked like a sanitorium or asylum did little to reassure the public. Virtually all HIV-infected patients in Melbourne were treated at Fairfield and so the other hospitals didn't become experienced in dealing with them. In the rest of the country, where there were no dedicated infectious diseases hospitals, HIV patients were a little more widely distributed, but most were still clustered in a handful of institutions.

The staff at Fairfield had lived through many epidemics and had been treating patients with potentially deadly transmissible infections for decades. This is not to say that they were complacent or oblivious to the risk, quite the opposite: they were keenly aware of the infectious dangers of medical practice, but they had created an environment where infection control was second nature – the prevention of transmission of pathogens from patient to staff or from patient to patient was built into the culture of the place. Everyone from the switchboard operators to the medical superintendent spoke the same language of infection prevention. But there was also a sense among the staff that the willingness to expose yourself to the risk made you a bit special – and indeed many of them were.

Away from Fairfield, however, there were dozens of examples coming to light of behaviour that could only be regarded as the antithesis of special. I can excuse the cleaners who were frightened of going into AIDS patients' rooms. I can sympathise with the food services people who would leave meals outside the doors. I can understand the ward clerks being hesitant in their dealings with patients. Such people were, in the main, acting out of ignorance rather than prejudice. But I can neither condone nor forgive the behaviour of a small but significant proportion of the medical profession who, because of either homophobia, moral outrage or fear for their personal safety, refused to see patients with HIV. They knew that the risks of transmission were actually very small. Some surgeons were refusing to see gay patients until they had an HIV test, and if it was positive many refused to operate on them. Some radiologists would not perform investigations that needed injections of contrast to make the images interpretable. There were gastroenterologists who wouldn't perform endoscopies, cardiologists who denied patients coronary angiograms. The list went on.

A pulchritudinous female orthopaedic surgeon from San Francisco appeared in the media spreading misinformation that HIV could be spread through droplets generated by the use of high-speed drills during operations. She argued that if it was in the air then everybody would need to wear space suits to avoid contagion. The evidence of the way HIV had been spreading for the previous five years showed this to be manifestly false, yet her ideas created doubt among the susceptible, coming as they did from a doctor working in one of the hotspots of the global HIV epidemic.

If you are going to catch HIV, the virus has to breach the skin or mucous membranes– this can happen through sex or through an accident with a contaminated sharp object such as a needle or scalpel. When I was a medical student it was almost a sport to see how many sharps you could fit in a disposal tin. My first exposure occurred when I was observing in the casualty department and I jabbed my finger on a needle that was sticking out of a jam-packed one-litre disposal tin. Up to then no one thought to empty the silly things before they overflowed. Once HIV arrived, new bins were designed and protocols for the safe disposal of sharp instruments were implemented. Dentists started to wear gloves and masks, surgeons changed their way of working when their hands were deep inside body cavities to reduce the chance of stabbing themselves (and their assistants), and the sterilisation of endoscopes and other objects that were inserted into people was intensified. The red of the bloodstains that were once worn as a badge of courage by young doctors came to be seen as a colour indicator of poor infection control.

Paradoxically, some doctors remained blasé bordering on indifferent when it came to some procedures involving sharp instruments. While some were worrying unnecessarily about things that carried little or no risk of transmission, others continued to do things in a way that defied belief. I knew of one pathologist who was exposed during an autopsy on a patient who had died of AIDS. Instead of cutting the viscera open on a solid surface, it was his habit to use a scalpel to slice open the organs while he held them in his left hand. One morning he stabbed the scalpel through both the liver he was examining and the palm of his hand.

Overall though, infection-control practices improved and it is likely that hundreds of thousands of non-HIV-infected patients inadvertently benefited as a result. The fear that the doctors felt for themselves was one reason why they improved their approach to asepsis and hygiene. But again, not everyone seemed to get it.

In 1994, more than ten years into the epidemic, four women contracted HIV in the rooms of a Sydney surgeon. The first patient on the surgeon's minor procedures list for the day was HIV positive, a fact not known by the patient or the surgeon at the time. Although never proved, it is believed that the bottle of local anaesthetic the surgeon was using had been contaminated by the first patient and was then used for each of subsequent women. Multi-dose vials of local anaesthetic were common despite the manifest risks, and it was only after this tragedy that the practice stopped – for a while at least *(see page 18)*.

Initially there was a call for testing of every patient being pre-pared for surgery – the main reason put forward being that this would allow the surgeon to be 'more careful' when he or she knew that the patient had HIV. There was a reasonably well-founded belief that the undeclared reason for the testing by some surgeons was to identify infected patients and to take them off waiting lists. Self-serving and ethical considerations aside, one of the main problems with the 'testing will protect us' approach is that you have to ask the question, testing for what? In 1988 there were antibody tests available for HIV and hepatitis B, but it would be another year until a test for hepatitis C – a virus about ten times more common in the population than HIV – became available. Then there are other viruses, such as HTLV-1 (human T-lympho-tropic virus type I, a cause of leukaemia and lymphoma in adults) which were far less common and rarely tested for. And it would be naive to believe that new human pathogens would not emerge in the future. The only way to protect yourself was to treat eve-ryone in exactly the same way, and if every patient received the same treatment, no one was being discriminated against.

I have noticed that over the past few years routine testing

has crept into contemporary surgical practice for elective procedures. This was once a contentious topic, with passionate arguments proposed from both sides, but pre-operative testing is more commonplace now and the increase has occurred without much public discussion. There are reports that there are some units that test all their patients pre-operatively for blood-borne viruses, and then refer them elsewhere if they are found to be positive for a viral infection. If this was their motivation for testing, not the welfare of their patients, the behaviour would be unethical. The irony is that with the availability of effective anti-viral medication for HIV there really *are* good reasons for testing patients in hospital. Because there are so many people with undiagnosed, and therefore untreated, HIV in the USA, the Centers for Disease Control now recommends all patients admitted to hospital have an HIV test so that they can be started on treatment before their immunosuppression is too far advanced. For HIV testing, as for so many things in medical practice, context and intention is everything.

Quantifying risk

The good news is that transmission of blood-borne viruses in a medical setting is an incredibly rare event. Although it is impossible to exactly determine the risk, you can estimate what the chances of someone contracting an infection are after an accidental exposure. The most dangerous type of needlestick is one which involves a hollow-bore needle – the sort used in injections – because it is more likely to have a small amount of a patient's blood left in it than a suture needle of the type I had used to sew Peter J's intercostal tube in place.

If a needle which has been used on a patient with one of the three common blood-borne viruses penetrates the skin of the person performing the procedure, the risks of transmission are usually quoted to be as follows: 0.3 per cent (or 3 in 1000 exposures) for HIV; 3 per cent for hepatitis C; and 30 per cent for hepatitis B. The reason that there is a roughly ten-fold difference in risk between the three viruses is that each has a different inherent degree of infectivity. Only a few copies of the hepatitis B virus can cause infection, while it takes a larger exposure to HIV to infect someone. The number of particles of a virus present in the bloodstream of a patient at any particular point in time is also an important factor in the risk of transmission. It is known that the number of HIV particles in a person's bloodstream is highest in the few months just after infection occurs and then drops off for many years until it rises again when the immune system has become profoundly depleted. Treatment with antiviral drugs can dramatically reduce the number of HIV particles in the blood, and so it is important to know whether the source patient in a needlestick incident is taking anti-HIV medication and what the viral load in his blood is at the time of the exposure. Some people have a natural resistance to HIV as a result of a mutation which is present on some of their white cells (this mutation is found in about 10 per cent of caucasians but is rare among African and southeast Asian populations – a genetic diversity that may partly explain the different patterns of spread of HIV across the globe). Other individuals are resistant to HIV for unknown reasons. Patients with hepatitis B are known to have different levels of infectivity depending on how much control their immune system has over the multiplication of the virus.

So while a guide to the average risk of transmission can be given, there are many things that will influence an individual's risk of contracting the infection from a needlestick incident. It is important to remember that the vast majority of such exposures occur where it is not known if the source patient actually has a viral infection. In Australia, less than 0.1 per cent of the population has HIV and around 0.5–1 per cent has hepatitis C.

So unless the source patient has a higher risk of being infected (is a gay man or comes from a country with high levels of HIV, say) you multiply the estimated prevalence of the virus in the community by the risk of transmission. For example, the risk of contracting HIV from a needlestick that involved a female Australian patient with no obvious risk factors is 0.3 per cent x 0.08 per cent, or a risk of around 1 in 416 666. The risk of catching hepatitis C under the same scenario would be 3 per cent x 1 per cent or 1 in 3333.

The protocol for follow-up of an occupational exposure usually involves blood tests at six weeks, three and six months after the event. For HIV, almost everyone who is going to become infected will do so within six weeks of exposure and the three-month test is really a formality. On the other hand, the incubation period for hepatitis B and C is much longer and you can't be confident until six months have elapsed. It is, believe me, a long semester.

Today, a person who receives a needlestick from a known HIV-positive patient would receive antiviral prophylaxis for four weeks. The drugs recommended are extremely safe, and while the benefit of prophylaxis is small (because the risk of contracting HIV *without* it is only 3 in 1000), it has become the standard of care. Hepatitis B is rarely a problem because almost all health care workers are vaccinated against it. If they are not, a high dose of anti-hepatitis B antibodies can be administered after the event, which is highly protective. It is hepatitis C that poses the biggest risk, because it is relatively common and there is no antiviral prophylaxis available. Recently it has been shown that if patients with hepatitis C are treated within 12 months of becoming infected, the chance of cure is extremely high. It is, therefore, a matter of 'wait-and-C'.

Prevention is better than cure

Three months passed after I stuck myself and it was time for my final HIV test. Ghosts of girlfriends-past visited me the night before. I relived every occupational exposure that I could recall, every time I had been covered in blood from 1980 onwards. I knew that the numbers were on my side, yet no matter how many times I soliloquised the arguments that I would use with my own patients, I couldn't convince myself of their truth. My test at six weeks was negative and, as a result, the chance of being infected had now dropped even further than the 3 in 1000 figure. When I pay my money for the office Tattslotto ticket I have no belief that I will win – the odds are just too low for me to raise any thrill of anticipation. Yet, a risk of even 1 in 10 000 seemed like a certainty before my blood was drawn.

The way we perceive risk is determined by the weight of the possible consequences. In 1989 the significance of contracting HIV was very different from what it would be today, when anti-viral drugs that completely suppress infection are available. I didn't share my fears with my wife, and, fortunately, with a new-born taking all our energies, there hadn't been an opportunity for transmission in our nappy-packed, sleepless and other-focused lives.

In 20 years of counselling people who have undergone occupational exposures I have never treated anyone who has contracted hepatitis C or HIV, and I have had only one who caught hepatitis B. The published literature confirms my personal experience of the rarity of transmission as a result of medical work. Needlesticks that occur in the community, away from the hospital environment, continue to intermittently attract media attention. I remember a news conference that was convened after a well known iron man competitor stuck himself on a syringe buried on a beach. Looking more marshmallow than ferrous, the poor guy was visibly disturbed and anxious as he spoke on-camera. He quoted the figures that he had been given for transmission risk that apply to the healthcare setting. His fears could have been allayed if his doctor had let him know that there has never been an HIV transmission from a needlestick in a non-medical setting in Australia – or, to my knowledge, anywhere else in the world.

Still, while the risk from needlestick incidents in the medical context is low, the anxiety and suffering can be enormous. Although some staff members take possible exposure to infection in their stride, most are affected in some way. At the extreme end, I have seen people leave their jobs, abandon their family, or become suicidal. The majority are distracted in their work and domestic lives. If the source patient is known then it is usually a relatively simple matter to obtain consent from him or her for testing: if the source's tests are negative, then there is virtually no risk of transmission. The only exception to this is if the patient is in the window period of infection. This is an extremely rare occurrence in Australia – although it has happened. In 1999 a ten-year-old girl in Melbourne contracted HIV from a blood transfusion which was negative for HIV antibodies. Soon after, a new testing technology was introduced that reduced the non-detectable period to about 11 days.

It goes without saying that prevention is better than cure. And because I have had to repeat this old chestnut here, it also goes without saying that some people don't take any notice of the adage. Every hospital has a unit dedicated to the prevention and management of occupational exposures – they try to reduce the number of exposures by instituting a safer workplace. They educate the staff about safe working practices and collect data to see how they are doing. The unit ensures that there are adequate disposal bins, that these are emptied regularly and that the hospital uses equipment which is inherently safe. (For example, intravenous cannulas are available that automatically place a protective shield over the needle when it is withdrawn from the patient's vein.) Some units do better than others at reducing the number of incidents that occur. The unit at my hospital has managed to maintain the annual number of incidents to between 100 and 150, and many of these – such as a splash of urine or saliva – are trivial, and carry virtually no risk of transmission. Yet despite what I would have thought is a major driver of safe practice – self-interest – I still watch colleagues and junior staff break the rules: interns who don't wear gloves when they insert intravenous cannulas ('I can't feel the vein' is a common excuse. My riposte is that microsurgeons can rejoin nerves as thin as a hair while they wear gloves, so get over it). Registrars and nurses who perform procedures where there is a risk of a splash often don't wear eye protection. Witnessed excuse: 'I don't look good in those goggles'. Even today, residents sometimes leave sharp instruments in trays after they have performed a procedure, or, even worse, allow the sharp to find its way into a linen disposal bag, where it then sticks a member of the cleaning staff. If only I could show these doctors and nurses how bad they will feel after they have sustained an occupational exposure. If only I could let them get a taste of the anguish before the event, experience just a little of the anxiety that a needlestick can generate.

Three months passed. Peter J made it out of intensive care but died in Ward 4 a few weeks later.

All my tests were negative.

5

Malcolm in the beginning

Clostridium tetani – a rod-shaped Gram-positive anaerobic
bacillus that sometimes appears like a tennis racket under the
microscope. The organism can produce spores that are resistant
to cold and heat, and can survive for long periods in soil and
organic material. Penetrating wounds contaminated with *C.
tetani* spores are said to be 'tetanus prone'. If conditions are right,
the organism starts to multiply in the wound and produces a
powerful nerve toxin. Patients with tetanus develop local muscle
rigidity, painful whole-body spasms and can choke to death
if the throat muscles are involved. Once a dreaded disease,
vaccination has almost completely eradicated tetanus from the
developing world.

'A mysterious new syndrome [has] emerged in the US:
thousands of children are developing AIDS symptoms (with
deranged T4 and T8 cells) without being HIV positive. My
well-considered opinion is that it comes from that T (standing
for tetanus) in the DPT vaccine.' (Dr Viera Scheibner, winner
of the 1997 Australian Skeptics Bent Spoon Award – presented
to individuals or organisations who made the most outrageous
claim of a paranormal or pseudoscientific nature in the
preceding year)

I did not fall in love with medicine until my third year at university, for it was then that we finally started on subjects that had attracted me to the profession in the first place – pathology, microbiology and pharmacology among them. Our main lecturer in microbiology was Jos Forsyth, a tall, ginger-haired man who looked a little like the Swedish chef from The Muppets. His course was based on a photocopied manual of lecture notes that catalogued all the microbes we were expected to know. Bound in an orange cover and known as the Tangerine Terror, it was essentially a textbook of microbiology pared down to bullet points. Students were expected to learn everything contained in it, and, at around 300 pages, this was a daunting task. For four lectures a week over 30 weeks, 220 of us sat in a cavernous lecture theatre and copied down everything that Jos said. Well, almost everything.

Sometimes he would pause and say something like: 'The next bit isn't examinable', and pens would be put down for a moment while he related an interesting but unessential piece of information. He was famous for his impersonation of a patient with whooping cough, an infection that then was fast becoming just a memory. His repetitive coughing, starting stertorously, then accelerating rapidly to culminate in the high-pitched whoop of indrawn breath, was met with rapturous applause. He would take a small bow and then make it clear that the next bit was indeed examinable.

I filled page after page of A4 ruled paper with the names of bacteria, the media that they would grow on, the types of sugar that they metabolised, what they looked like under the microscope and what antibiotics they were sensitive to. At the end of the first week I was dazzled by the range of organisms in existence and I rejoiced in the wonder of their varied biologies. By the end of the second week I was starting to wonder if I would be able to remember all their names and properties. By the close of the third week, with 12 lectures already in my folder I was starting to curse biodiversity, and care less and less about microbes as individuals. By the fourth week I was completely pissed off with microbiology and Jos Forsyth's phonebook approach to teaching.

In addition, we had to know all the drugs in Goodman and Gilman's *Manual of Pharmacology and Therapeutics*, the bible on the subject. I had the feeling that my brain was beginning to fill up and I started justifying my inadequacy by questioning the relevance of what I was learning. But then tutorials with Malcolm started.

Breathing life into learning

I was living at Ormond College at the time and one of the benefits of staying on campus was the extra tutorials that were offered. I had managed to avoid almost all of them the previous year but after I escaped the ignominy of failing biochemistry by a margin of just three marks, I realised that I needed to take things a little more seriously. Malcolm McDonald was a medical registrar from the Royal Melbourne Hospital who was training to be an infectious diseases specialist. His supervisor had advised him to become a tutor because he knew that you really only come to understand a topic when you have been able to teach it to someone else. His tutorials were held in a room furnished with wooden desks that were nearly 100 years old, and the board was black, not white. The use of an overhead projector was seen as a bit avant garde in the late 1970s and any tutor who brought colour slides to a tutorial was obviously an authority. Malcolm did neither. He would just sit on the edge of the desk at the front of the room and tell us stories, which would often start with a question.

What had we been hearing about in the lectures that week, he asked. When one of us told him syphilis, he smiled and asked if you could catch it from a toilet seat. We looked around at each other, slightly bemused.

'The treponeme is an extremely delicate organism that has caused dreadful damage to the brains, hearts and cartilage of thousands of young, and not-so-young lovers', he said. 'It knows no social boundaries and can be found in every street of every town in this country. But it can't be caught from a toilet seat. Yet when I was a student my father told me, "It doesn't matter if you stand on the seat, the spirochaete can jump six feet".'

He looked at the group of 19 year olds in front of him who were now starting to smile. 'I am afraid gentlemen that there is only one way to contract syphilis and that is through the act of love and its variations, including fellatio and cunnilingus. The latter is not named after the Irish airline by the way.'

We were all laughing by now and I settled back into my chair with the dawning realisation that I had a found a way to learn the names of thousands of germs and their quirks and proclivities: Malcolm was going to give us something precious to hang our isolated pieces of knowledge onto – clinical anecdotes.

The following week we met the anaerobic bacterium *Clostridium tetani* – the cause of tetanus. Tetanus is a vanishingly rare disease in Australia, not because of improving living standards or diet but simply because of the near universality of vaccination that began in the 1920s. During the Second World War all Australian servicemen were vaccinated against tetanus and not a single case of it occurred, something unheard of in the history of warfare. Mass vaccination against the disease became an accepted part of the public health system by the 1950s, and to this group of third-years born in the 1960s tetanus seemed a historical curiosity.

'Do you know the story about the night cart worker from Numurkah?' Malcolm asked. Numurkah is a small town on the Murray River about two and a half hours' drive north of Melbourne, and in the 1970s it still wasn't completely sewered. Many households had outhouses for their daily ablutions and each night a truck (the night cart) would take away the 'night soil'. The night cart worker, Malcolm told us, woke one morning late in September feeling a little unwell. He noticed that he was having difficulty opening his mouth, a problem that got worse as the day went on. His GP examined him, diagnosed a tooth abscess and prescribed antibiotic capsules. The man took a first capsule that evening, but next morning was unable to open his mouth at all and his teeth were involuntarily clenched together. His wife remarked on his smug expression. It was AFL grand final day in Victoria and he had tickets to the MCG and wouldn't miss the game for anything. He drove to Melbourne and bought a can of beer at the ground, forgetting he couldn't drink. Then he realised that he could put the gap left by his missing front teeth to good purpose. He obtained a straw and sucked one of the antibiotic capsules through it, followed by a draught of beer. But he was now having difficulty swallowing even his own saliva. The capsule sat on his tongue, the outer gelatin dissolving in the beer and releasing the antibiotic powder. The combination of antibiotic and carbonated drink resulted in an effervescent eruption in his mouth and the man from Numurkah started to choke, just as the ball was bounced for the first quarter. He collapsed, a St John Ambulance lady arrived and he was carried off to the Royal Melbourne Hospital, where he was diagnosed with tetanus.

Throughout the telling, Malcolm mimicked the appearance of the night cart man, his face becoming tighter and tighter as he acted out the story. His voice developed the high-pitched tenor of the patient who is losing control of his facial and swallowing muscles, and he demonstrated to us what is known as *risus sardonicus* – the ironic grin of the patient with tetanus. His timing was impeccable and we were all laughing so loudly that a couple of students in the tutorial group next door came in to see what the fuss was all about. We spent the rest of the session revising the microbiology of *C. tetani* and discussing its treatment and prevention.

Malcolm lacked any qualifications in education, had never

heard of a learning agreement and would have baulked at some of the ideas of modern educational theory, but he was able to inspire in his students the same love for the subject that he had himself.

'And that', he said just before dismissing us, 'was the very first patient I saw on my first day as a doctor'.

How vaccination vanquished tetanus

The injection of tetanus toxoid into people after a penetrating injury has been such a reflex action by nurses and doctors for half a century that the disease has almost been completely eradicated in the developed world. In fact, by the 1980s people were receiving tetanus vaccinations too often – many of them were needless (although none were needle-less). The ache and tenderness that you feel in your arm after a tetanus shot signifies that you are making a very good immune response to it, indeed the stronger the reaction the less likely the need to have had the booster in the first place because you already had immunity from previous vaccination. The guidelines now recommend that if you have received a proper course of tetanus vaccination as a child and young adult, a booster is not needed until you are 50 years old, and none after that unless you sustain a tetanus-prone wound. Tetanus was once dreaded in the general community. Before the vaccination of the population, hundreds of patients would be admitted to Australian hospitals each year; by 2008 only four cases were diagnosed across the country.

C. tetani lives in the environment in the form of spores. Spores are hardy, non-multiplying forms of the bacterium that can live in the soil for years and can survive extremes of heat and cold. Once they get into a more hospitable place – a human wound, for example – they change into growing bacteria which release a toxin that invades the nerves, progressively affecting more and more of the body. The toxin makes the nerves extremely irritable and a trivial stimulus that they would normally ignore becomes a major trigger for action: the nerves fire off and cause contraction of the muscles that they are connected to. The prolonged, so-called tetanic contraction, causes the intensely painful and distressing muscle spasms that are characteristic of the disease. Once the toxin has been produced, treatment with penicillin only stops more growth of the bacteria and has no effect on the toxin itself. Reversal of the effect of the toxin requires the injection of a high dose of anti-toxin antibodies. Before the development of intensive care units and the routine use of ventilators to maintain the breathing of unconscious patients, someone with tetanus would be heavily sedated and nursed on a general ward. The patient would have a chance of survival if the disease had not progressed to involve the respiratory and swallowing muscles, and if the anti-toxin had been administered early enough. The family and the nursing staff would then have to watch the patient suffer through days, weeks and even months of spasms that could affect the whole body, or sometimes just the muscles of the throat. The spasms might come on at any time, sometimes literally at the drop of a hat, or other similarly innocent trigger. (My father remembered a sign outside St Vincent's Hospital in Melbourne in the 1950s that asked drivers not to sound their horn because of tetanus patients inside.)

More than half the patients would die. Survival was a tribute to meticulous nursing care. I have only been directly involved in the treatment of four cases of tetanus – one when I was a student in India, involving a boy whose symptoms included opisthotonus (where the spinal muscles contract and the body arches in spasm so that only the back of the head and the feet are touching the bed). It is something that I do not wish to see again. The other three tetanus cases were in Australia and much less dramatic because the patients were intubated, artificially paralysed and sedated. The muscle spasms are prevented by the administration of curare-like drugs (the plant toxin used by South American Indians to paralyse hunted animals) which stop the nerves from firing, and, in addition, the patients are maintained in a pharmacological haze. All three patients were gardeners in late middle age who had never received a primary course of vaccination. All survived after months in the intensive care unit.

There is no 'natural' immunity to tetanus – only vaccination protects you. The three gardeners still needed a full course of vaccination after recovery or they would have been at risk of contracting tetanus again: while extremely rare, there are documented cases of this microbiological lightning striking twice.

In the aftermath of the 2004 Boxing Day tsunami, over 100 cases of tetanus were diagnosed among survivors in the Sumatran city of Banda Aceh. The mainly unvaccinated population were exposed to the bacterial spores when they sustained cuts and abrasions in the tidal wave and floods, and with an average incubation period of just over a week, the disease flowed as the waters ebbed. Generally, however, tetanus is a disease of the newborn in the developing world – babies being exposed at the time of birth. If the mother has been vaccinated, protective antibodies are passed across the placenta to the baby, but the babies of unvaccinated women have no such protection.

The limits of protection in the herd

Tetanus is different from most infectious diseases because there is no herd immunity associated with it. Herd immunity is the concept that a group will be protected from infection once a certain proportion of the whole population has been immunised, either by catching the infection or being vaccinated against it. The necessary proportion varies according to the disease – the more contagious the pathogen is, the higher the proportion must be to afford protection to the rest. For example, the global eradication of smallpox, with the exception of some samples of the virus held in laboratories in Russia and the USA, was facilitated by two biological properties of the virus: a lower level of infectivity than some other infectious diseases, and the fact that the virus can only be passed between humans – there was no animal reservoir. These characteristics made it possible to remove the disease from the face of the earth by vaccinating people who lived close to smallpox cases. Once outbreaks of smallpox had been isolated in this way, the disease disappeared. Global eradication has not been achieved for any other communicable diseases, although the end of polio is tantalisingly close. For some diseases, eradication may never be possible. Measles, for example, is so infectious that a minimum of 95 per cent of the population must be immunised to develop herd immunity for the remaining 5 per cent, and since the vaccine is only 95 per cent effective it will be almost impossible to achieve this – eradication will have to wait until a more effective vaccine is developed.

Herd immunity is the main thing that protects children whose parents do not vaccinate them. But populations are never static: babies are born, people die and migrate in and out – so that the number of susceptible people keeps changing and eventually reaches the critical level where a disease can reappear in the population. The cyclical nature of measles epidemics in a number of islands in the Pacific demonstrates this.

It is understandable that young women who have been brought up by mothers without first-hand experience of any of the classical childhood illnesses that can kill children may be influenced by the carefully crafted, but intellectually flawed (and sometimes even dishonest) arguments of the anti-vaccination movement. I remember when my first child received her initial set of vaccines I felt the needle go into her leg as though it were mine, and I worried about her for the rest of the day and through the night. Although I had seen children nearly choking to death from whooping cough, cared for polio patients who were still living in their iron lungs nearly 40 years after they contracted the disease, and seen tetanus kill that young man in India, my mind travelled straight to the incredibly rare risks that vaccines pose. If someone like me hesitates, is it any wonder that others who haven't spent much of their life thinking about infectious diseases would have doubts and fears?

These misgivings about vaccines are fuelled by several incidents. In 1927, 12 Australian children died in what became known as the Bundaberg disaster. A dose of diphtheria vaccine had been kept at room temperature by one of the local medical officers. This had allowed bacterial contaminants to grow in the vial, which did not contain a preservative. The inoculated children developed a toxic shock-like illness caused by *Staphylococcus aureus* (see chapter 7). A worse incident occurred in 1955 when a batch of one of the earliest versions of the polio vaccine was inadequately inactivated and over 100 recipients developed polio as a consequence; around a dozen of them died. Such was the fear of diphtheria and polio among parents, however, that vaccination uptake was restored once it was shown that the problem was confined to one vial in the case of the diphtheria deaths and a single batch of vaccine in the case of the polio victims.

In 1976 a vaccine against swine flu was associated with an increase in the occurrence of a neurological condition called Guillain-Barré syndrome *(see page 15)*. The vaccine-associated risk was around eight cases per million people vaccinated, which was similar to the background risk for the disease in the general population, but because the swine flu epidemic did not eventuate, the vaccine-related cases of Guillain-Barré syndrome were not balanced by hundreds of swine flu-associated cases among the unvaccinated population.

Vaccination, it has been said, is the single most cost-effective medical intervention of the past 100 years. It has saved, prolonged and improved the quality of millions, possibly billions, of lives. But to achieve this a small, but not trivial, number of recipients will experience adverse reactions that range from a sore arm, to a fever and allergic reaction, all the way to death. This is the burden of every parent who consents to their child being vaccinated, and every health professional who advocates vaccination. A thousand prevented cases of an infection are invisible; a single, serious consequence of vaccination stays etched in the public consciousness for years. The social contract for vaccination between the public and health authorities is delicate: it can be broken at any time and so needs nurturing and maintenance. But a world without vaccines would not be a safer one and those who think it would be, misinterpret and misrepresent history, epidemiology and common sense.

Unfortunately too many children have reaped the harvest of our hesitations. And what a bumper crop it has been for some diseases: the plummeting rate of whooping cough vaccination in the 1980s because of unfounded fears of irreversible neurological side-effects led to a return of the disease and of the terrors of nursing tiny babies who coughed themselves blue and turned their parents white. Many died as a result. Then there was the scurrilous proposal by a British doctor that the MMR (measles, mumps and rubella) vaccine was associated with autism. The scare allowed an 18th century disease to enjoy a 21st century return season.

A cohort of middle-class, cosseted, non-immunised children are now getting to be old enough to travel to the developing world, where communicable diseases still rule. I can imagine their surprise when they contract an illness that a vaccine would have protected them against. I anticipate that their parents, sincere but ignorant to the end, will search vainly for homeopathic remedies for the diseases that their homeopathic 'vaccines' failed to prevent. I wonder how they will deal with the look of disappointment in their children's eyes when they face them on their return. If they do return, that is.

6

The Semmelweis effect

Streptococcus pyogenes – a Gram-positive coccus that appears as chains of blue dots under the microscope. Also known as Group A streptococcus, the organism can change from peaceful coloniser of the throat of its human hosts to aggressive invader of the deep tissues and muscles. In the 19th century it was the commonest cause of puerperal fever, a major killer of women after giving birth. Some strains produce a toxin which, among other things, causes rheumatic fever and necrotising fasciitis – the so-called flesh-eating disease – a condition that can progress rapidly. Despite its potential to cause some of the most deadly human bacterial infections, *S. pyogenes* is always sensitive to penicillin.

'What, will these hands ne'er be clean?' (from *Macbeth*, by William Shakespeare, 1564–1616)

On 30 July 1865, at the age of only 47, Ignaz Semmelweis, the Hungarian father of hand hygiene, was committed to a Viennese asylum. He had deteriorated mentally over the preceding years, to the point where associates tricked him into visiting the institution under the pretence that he was on an inspection tour, then had him incarcerated. Semmelweis had become increasingly obsessed with his ideas about hand hygiene, which had been rejected by the mainstream European medical community. Most of his colleagues ignored his observations and experimental data demonstrating that the use of a chlorinated hand-wash could prevent the transmission of puerperal fever (childbed fever) from one woman to another on the hands of medical attendants. The English said his findings were nothing new, and the German doyen of modern pathology, Rudolph Virchow, rejected Semmelweis's claims outright. He responded with open letters, accusing the medical establishment of being murderers for failing to take heed of his recommendations on hand disinfection. Before his incarceration, Semmelweis had taken to drink and been seen carousing around town with prostitutes. While popular folklore holds that it was the establishment's rejection of his ideas despite the evidence (what has come to be called the Semmelweis effect) that drove him mad, the underlying cause of his cognitive decline is not clear. Early-onset Alzheimer's disease or tertiary syphilis have been suggested as reasons.

While trying to escape from his enforced hospitalisation Semmelweis was beaten by the guards and as a result developed a gangrenous leg wound. Two weeks later he was dead. His post-mortem suggested that he had died of pyaemia (blood poisoning). We will never know which bug killed him because it would be another 20 years before Robert Koch would confirm the germ theory of disease and teach the world how to associate individual pathogens with specific conditions. It would not, however, be too fanciful to suggest that Semmelweis succumbed to an infection caused by the same bacterium that was the main cause of the disease he had spent his life working on.

In 1846 Semmelweis was appointed as First Assistant at the First Obstetric Clinic at the Vienna General Hospital. This clinic was established to provide obstetric training for medical students and, as part of the emerging positivist philosophy of German medicine, the relationship between structure and function, cause and effect was assiduously explored. If a woman died in childbirth or soon after, she would undergo a post-mortem examination, often performed by the same doctor or medical student who was involved in the delivery. Although the figures fluctuated throughout the year, the average death rate from puerperal sepsis in the First Clinic was around 13 per cent. Semmelweis observed that the death rate at the Second Obstetric Clinic, which was for the instruction of midwives only (they took no part in post-mortems) was just 2 per cent. He proposed that 'cadaverous matter' was being transferred from the post-mortem room to living mothers on the hands of the medical students and doctors in the First Clinic. If he was right, hand-cleaning should reduce the death rate. The results of a regimen of hand hygiene emphatically suggested Semmelweis was right: the death rate in the First Clinic fell to 2 per cent within a month of the introduction of chlorinated lime hand-washing. The practice was resisted by the staff – chlorinated lime is hard on the skin and it is likely that they complained about the effect it was having on their hands.

The germ theory of disease transmission may have been proved by Koch and Pasteur, but it had been widely understood that disease could be spread from one patient to another since ancient times. The problem was that the actual means of transmission of disease was not understood. Some larger micro-organisms could be seen with the earliest microscopes – Van Leeuwenhoek described mouth bacteria in 1674 – but the quality of optics was inadequate to resolve most bacteria until the 19th century, and it would not be until the development of special staining techniques by the Danish bacteriologist Hans Christian Gram that the clear identification of specific bacteria would be possible.

Semmelweis did not know that bacteria were causing puerperal sepsis, but he did know that removing putrid matter from the hands of birth attendants before they examined a woman in labour reduced her chance of dying by a factor of at least three.

Some critics argued that there would be inadequate material on the hands of attendants to cause disease – they took a strictly 'chemical' approach to contagion, which would be supplanted a few decades later when it was realised that bacteria could multiply rapidly when the conditions were right.

A killer in the blood

We now understand that the commonest cause of puerperal sepsis is the bacterium *Streptococcus pyogenes*. There are dozens of streptococci that cause human disease, including Group B strep infections, which are the most common bacterial cause of neonatal illness among new mothers in the developed world today. Infection is rarely serious, and since up to 25 per cent of women carry Group B strep in their vaginas the illness is not caused by cross-infection. Other bacteria, such as *Staphylococcus aureus* (see chapter 7), are also implicated in neonatal illness, but are very rare.

But *S. pyogenes*, also called Group A strep, is much more potent. Under the microscope it appears as little dots (cocci) that form into short chains which are purple when Gram-stained. It is differentiated from other streptococci by its ability to break down the red blood cells on the agar plates it is grown on. It can cause many distinct diseases – it is the commonest bacterial cause of tonsillitis and, if a particular strain is responsible, rheumatic fever may follow. Skin sores are common manifestations of infection and, in some cases, post-infective inflammation of the kidney can ensue.

Pyogenes means 'pus forming', and this is one of the hallmarks of Group A strep. Pus is a mixture of white blood cells, dead human tissue cells, serum and the bacteria themselves. It is the immune system of the infected person that produces the pus: the presence of the multiplying bacteria triggers a local response, with white blood cells recruited to the site of infection to destroy the invading organisms. One group of white blood cells, called neutrophils, produce enzymes and other chemicals which break down the bacteria, which are then literally eaten by another type of white blood cell, called macrophages (from the Greek, meaning 'big eaters'). The surrounding tissue can be collateral damage in this immunological blitzkrieg. Group A strep infection can result in abscesses anywhere in the body, but the head and neck are the commonest sites. And if the bug escapes from the abscess into the bloodstream, the infected patient becomes very sick indeed.

The ability of Group A strep to produce a powerful toxin adds weight to its infective punch. For unknown reasons, some strains in some people can invade the skin through an often trivial wound and then move into the deeper tissues between the muscles and start to multiply at a prodigious rate. The toxin produced in the process accelerates the breakdown of the tissue. This is the disease necrotising fasciitis – what the media calls 'the flesh-eating bug'. I have watched necrotising fasciitis rapidly move up a patient's thigh to involve the skin and deeper tissues of the groin, abdomen and back. Although it is an exaggeration to say that you can watch it spread in front of your eyes, there is undoubtedly detectable movement over a very short interval of time. Without intensive care, antibiotics and urgent surgery, someone with necrotising fasciitis will certainly die.

Some strains of Group A strep produce a toxin that results in the once common disease, scarlet fever, which can be a complication of a simple streptococcal throat infection or be associated with infections after surgery. The toxin affects the entire body and, depending on the amount of the toxin produced, scarlet fever can range from mild to deadly. People with the disease develop a sunburn-like rash, hence the name, and a 'strawberry tongue'. The function of the kidneys, lungs and liver can be impaired, and in its most serious manifestation the heart can fail. My mother suffered a mild attack of scarlet fever as a child in the 1920s. She survived (of course) but her favourite teddy bear, considered to be contaminated, didn't. It was cremated.

Scarlet fever virtually disappeared from the western world in the 1950s but in the late 1970s a scarlet fever-like illness called toxic shock syndrome started to emerge in menstruating women who were not replacing tampons frequently enough. Here, the toxin was produced by *Staph. aureus,* which was multiplying in the tampons, not Group A strep, but the clinical picture was identical to scarlet fever symptoms.

Group A strep has never developed resistance to penicillin, but don't let that provide you with too much comfort. I have seen the pathogen kill fit, young people within 48 hours, despite the administration of appropriate antibiotics.

The risks of rule-breaking

I can identify with Semmelweis's frustration and impatience with the prevailing professional attitude towards antisepsis. I am constantly amazed by the insouciance of my colleagues when it comes to infection control. Although they would never admit it, I suspect that the availability of antibiotics encourages a form of moral hazard in regard to prevention of transmission. In the pre-antibiotic era there was a clear relationship between an infection and the risk of death. The current laissez-faire approach to hand hygiene would not have been tolerated in a hospital in 1935, when it was well known by the most lowly medical officer that the development of a trivial hospital-acquired infection could kill a patient. That is still the case, of course, but many modern (and lofty) medical practitioners seem oblivious to the fact. It is as if these latter-day Doubting Thomases have inspected their hands and, failing to see the stigmata, do not believe in the infection. I have suggested, in moments of what observers have incorrectly assumed to be levity, that some of my colleagues have not quite realised that germs are small – I mean really, really small. So small you can only see them with a microscope. I imagine them asking, just as Semmelweis's critics did, how could something so tiny cause so much mayhem?

A surgeon arrives for an early morning ward round with registrar and resident in tow. A first-year medical student is there too, conducting a piece of discrete research for the infection control unit. The group walks into the room of the first patient, accompanied by the charge nurse of the ward, and exchange superficial pleasantries with the patient.

'Good morning, you're looking better', the patient is told. He has a tube in his stomach, via his nose, and is wearing an oxygen mask. 'Uhm ogay, thanggs', says the patient. The surgeon looks at the operation wound on the man's belly, feels his abdomen, checking for tenderness, and, with a quick and pleasant wave goodbye, leaves the room.

The next patient is a woman and she is a little sicker. Again the abdomen is palpated and the wound checked. There is an area of redness around the edges of the incision and, as pressure is applied, a small amount of pus is expressed from the wound. 'Better put her on some antibiotics', the surgeon tells the registrar, and is out the door before the resident can finish writing up the drugs on the medication chart.

Then to the next room and a third post-operative patient: another examination is performed, but this time everything is fine. The group finishes the round with a discussion of the theatre list for the next day. The surgeon retrieves her handbag from the work station and, with a courteous nod in the direction of the charge nurse, she leaves the ward.

The medical student's task was to observe how many times the team disinfected their hands between patients. The modern approach to hand hygiene does not require individuals to wash their hands with soap and water after every patient contact.

There is now overwhelming evidence that solutions containing a mixture of alcohol and chlorhexidine (a disinfectant) kill more germs more quickly than soap and water, and cause less irritation and dermatitis of the hands. Soap and water are still used to remove obvious soiling of the hands and is recommended after every 30 minutes or so of continuous patient contact. The student's report shows that no one disinfected their hands before or after contact with any of the three patients. A similar report from another student shows that the nursing staff were better in their hand-hygiene compliance, but even this group failed to follow the rules on at least 30 per cent of occasions.

Things are different in the operating theatre, though. While a nurse from a former generation would be horrified by the sight of anaesthetists and surgeons eating and drinking in the anterooms, and at the mess that can exist on benches and in corridors, asepsis is alive and well in the modern operating theatre, at least during the operation itself. There is an almost religious devotion to the ritual of hand-washing, sterility and the avoidance of contamination during an operation. But when the big lights are turned off and the performance is over, the surgeon, now out of costume and back in street clothes, will usually ignore the infection control policies of the rest of the hospital that they themselves would enforce in the operating theatre.

Papers can be presented at international meetings and appear in *The Lancet*, a dozen infection-control nurses can heave collective sighs of resigned disgust, *60 Minutes* can air an item on prime-time television, even the prime minister at the time of the 2009 swine flu pandemic can give advice focused on hand hygiene, but still too few people at the medical coalface appear to take note of the simple fact that if you disinfect your hands between patients the transmission of germs decreases dramatically and the rate of hospital-acquired infections falls accordingly. A patient may have had thousands of dollars' worth of anaesthetic drugs, drapes, instruments, clips and prostheses used in the course of an operation, but for the sake of a few cents' worth of alcohol and chlorhexidine hand disinfectant they are post-operatively exposed to the risk of hospital infection.

Claim and blame

Identifying the extent of the problem is the easy part, and many medical professionals are sick of reading about the poor level of adherence to the hygiene recommendations. The interested layperson, on the other hand, may be more concerned with the 'whys' rather than the 'whats', and would have many questions to ask the student who recorded the failure of consultant, registrar, resident and nurse to follow the rules on hand hygiene. Why, for example, didn't the nurse or the resident on the ward round speak up?

In previous times the ward was a nursing domain and what nurses said, went. Now there is a faux democracy in the workplace, facilitated by a generation of health workers that eschews hierarchy and authority – resulting often in a plethora of policy but a drought of practice. The impasse between medical and nursing staff is no longer a gender issue, more a result of the cultural and industrial divide that exists between the professional groups. The power differential between senior and junior medical personnel is profound, and it is a brave resident who pulls up a boss and tells them to disinfect their hands, especially if that resident is seeking preferment for scarce training positions.

Why didn't the patient say something? If there is a gradient between consultant and resident, and between resident and nurse, then the patient hasn't even reached base camp. A sense of powerlessness descends upon patients in hospital who in their home environment might be strong and outspoken. To suggest that the answer is to 'empower' them is unrealistic (test this the next time you are at the dentist: just before the drill starts spinning ask him how he sterilises his instruments).

Why isn't there a hospital policy about hand hygiene? There always is – but, like speed limits, it only works when it is enforced and potential offenders perceive that there is a high likelihood of being caught if they break the rules. There is no mechanism in place in most hospitals to ensure that hand antisepsis is adhered to, and if there was what punishments could be meted out to those failing to adhere to it? Why aren't students taught about hand hygiene in medical school? They are – students at our university know that they will fail their practical examinations if they don't disinfect their hands before and after they enter the examination room, but as soon as they enter a hospital where these rules are flouted by the nurses and doctors who provide their 'real education' they are soon acculturated. There is now a federally funded National Hand Hygiene initiative (part of a larger WHO plan) which is being rolled out across Australia – it is an overdue program that finally puts the issue on the national agenda. Education of the people responsible for the transmission of the germs is an essential first step, but adoption of hand antisepsis is often thwarted by the intransigence of senior and influential clinicians. Often, but not always.

Perhaps more than any other surgical group, orthopaedic surgeons are aware of the disaster that infection can spell and they go to great lengths to prevent it. If a patient develops an infection in a new prosthetic joint, the suffering can be severe.(Just how severe is highlighted by a study at the Canberra Hospital in which 12 per cent of patients being treated for infections after joint replacements rated their experience on a quality of life scale as being worse than death.) The monetary costs of an infected prosthesis are also severe. Surgeons earn more money from operating than from consulting – time spent in the wards mopping up the consequences of an infection is time lost in theatre. But perhaps more important than any other driver is the desire of orthopaedic surgeons to avoid having to do something which many of them are, by their own admission, constitutionally unsuited to

– having to talk to the same patient intermittently for months or even years. And even if they have the option of remedying things by doing what they love to do – operate – they are faced with a difficult and prolonged procedure: a joint replacement revision.

For these reasons, orthopaedic surgeons take additional precautions when they operate to prevent their patients from becoming infected. They wear two sets of gloves, protective suits that cover them from head to toe, and their theatres have what is known as laminar-flow air circulation to reduce the chance of stray environmental bacteria landing on the operative field. They ensure that intravenous antibiotics are administered during the induction of anaesthesia and become very nervous if a patient's operation wound shows any sign of redness or swelling. (Indeed, they can even over-react: some orthopaedic surgeons recommend that joint-replacement recipients take prophylactic antibiotics when they go to the dentist – something which is appropriate for people with an artificial heart valve but unnecessary, and probably ineffective, for people with artificial joints.)

Because the procedures are almost always elective, recipients of artificial joints tend to be more upset if they get infected in hospital. They express this distress in a number of ways: the most extreme and, fortunately, rare manifestation of their displeasure being litigation. In contrast, the relationship between cause and effect may not be so obvious in other areas of surgery. The patient who presents with, say, an inflamed appendix must have it removed – there is virtually no option. If they develop an infection after the operation then they tend to see it as a consequence of the appendicitis. However, a significant proportion of post-surgical infections have little to do with the underlying condition and more to do with the operation and other hospital procedures, such as an intravenous cannula or a urinary catheter that has been left in too long *(see chapter 7)*. The patient recovering from appendicectomy who develops a wound infection caused by MRSA (Methicillin-resistant *Staphylococcus aureus*) almost certainly caught it from another patient or someone on the hospital staff.

I worked with a surgeon in a regional hospital who was renowned for his technical acumen and ability to do just about anything. Since there was no vascular surgeon within 3000 kilometres, he had been called in to perform an emergency operation on someone with a leaking abdominal aortic aneurysm – the condition that killed Albert Einstein. The patient made a remarkable recovery, but a wound infection developed a week after the procedure and the patient was not happy. During the early morning ward round he told the surgeon that he was very displeased that the infection was delaying his discharge from hospital. 'A wound infection?' snapped the surgeon. 'I saved your fucking life. Be grateful.'

A case of mea culpa

Time to give my surgical colleagues a rest, for my own physicianly house is not in order. Nearly ten years ago my infection-control colleagues and my registrar conducted a small trial called Operation Stethoscope. We took swabs from the hands and stethoscopes of 134 members of our hospital staff. We found that 8 per cent of them grew *Staph aureus* on their hands and 4 per cent of the stethoscopes were contaminated with the same bacterium This was not rocket science, just a clear demonstration that the stethoscope around a doctor's (or nurse's or physiotherapist's) neck was an important potential source of cross-infection. I am embarrassed to admit that it came as a bit of a revelation to me at the time, but it forever changed my practise: I started to clean my stethoscope with an alcohol-impregnated swab after every use – something that disinfected it instantly. I did this with some ostentation when on a ward round: here is the boss leading the way, I reasoned. This will change collective behaviour, provide the kind of leadership that is so obviously needed. I discussed it with my colleagues and we agreed that in addition to an evangelical campaign to promote hand hygiene, cleaning of stethoscopes would become our standard operating procedure. We also placed a dispenser of alcohol/chlorhexidine hand-rub at the end of every bed in the hospital, outside every room and on every trolley. We changed the environment to make it easy to comply with hand hygiene rules between patients – and we encountered a deal of opposition. Here are some of the reasons why people have tried to stop us making the alcohol/chlorhexidine solution readily available: 'it is a dangerous good' (no it isn't); 'my hands will dry out' (no they won't – it is better than washing with soap and water); 'people will bump their shins on the brackets' (only if they are as tall as Michael Jordan); 'children will drink it' (taste it and see how much they can drink – think of sculling concentrated bubble bath); 'the mounting brackets will ruin the beds' (two screw holes are required); 'it's a fire hazard' (and the oxygen pouring out of the tube in the patient's nose isn't?).

Dozens of residents and registrars have rotated through our unit since these hygiene measures were introduced, yet apart from those who have chosen infectious diseases as their specialty, I cannot remember seeing any of them cleaning a stethoscope between patients once they have left our unit. Microbiological cultures, it appears, are much easier to modify than professional cultures.

I can see where one (unfortunate) part of the answer to the problem of non-compliance with infection-control procedures may lie. In the case of hand hygiene all but one of the elements in the equation have been attended to: we have formulated the rules (through countless hospital policies), modified the environment (alcohol/chlorhexidine hand-rub is widely available), and increased the receptivity of the players (educating medical and nursing staff, most recently through the National Hand Hygiene Initiative). Only an effective enforcement arm is lacking. But once it becomes plain to the patient population in general that there is a clear link between the behaviour of their medical attendants and the risk of them contracting an infection while in hospital, it is only going to take one high-profile case of a patient successfully suing a hospital for the climate on hygiene to change. Once a legal precedent has been set, the cost of a hospital-acquired infection to the health system will be directly measurable in litigation expenses and pay-outs, not hidden, as it currently is, in the day-to-day expenses associated with re-admission and prolonged hospital stays. When that happens we will see the rules truly put into force by those in control of the budgets.

And how then will the infection control community support their medical and nursing colleagues who have broken the rules? I could be wrong, but I think they will probably wash their hands of them.

7

In the blood

Staphylococcus aureus – a Gram-positive coccus that grows
in clusters. Popularly known as golden staph, it is one of the
commonest causes of bacterial infection in humans, affecting
the skin, muscles, bones, joints, brain and heart valves.
Resistance to penicillin was first observed in the 1950s, and an
increasing number of infections in the community are caused
by strains that are resistant to standard antibiotics. In hospital,
multi-resistant strains are an important cause of post-operative
complications. *S. aureus* infection of the bloodstream is a life-
threatening illness.

'Slowly the poison the whole blood stream fills. It is not
the effort nor the failure tire. The waste remains, the waste
remains and kills.' (from *Missing Dates*, by William Empson,
1906–1984)

The elite world of taxonomic microbiologists who get to decide
what we call our microscopic friends is divided into the 'lumpers'
and the 'splitters'. The lumpers try to minimise the number of
families and genuses that bacteria, viruses and other pathogens
can be scientifically classified into, while the splitters rejoice in
discovering subtle and minor differences between micro-organisms, and love to distinguish them as new species or occasionally

to create a new genus. Even as a practising infectious diseases specialist I have trouble keeping up with the names of bugs: every month or so our laboratory sends me a report which names a pathogen that I have never heard of. At the time of writing this, the most recent was *Nesterenkonia halobia*. I had to ask a colleague what it was.

'Used to be a micrococcus', she said. 'At least I could spell that.'

There is a degree of hypocrisy in this complaint, for I myself belong to a research group which changed the name of a bug (*see chapter 11*). In my defence, however, we showed that our germ belonged to an established genus, one whose properties – and spelling – were well known to the mainstream microbiological world. We brought our little charge in from the obscurity and loneliness of an unpronounceable genus – it was the sole species of the genus *Calymmatobacter* –and added it to a warm and loving family, the *Klebsiellae*.

But my pedantic taxonomic colleagues seem to delight in taking a relatively well known bug and, through a process reminiscent of Winston Smith in George Orwell's novel *Nineteen Eighty-Four*, depriving it of identity with the stroke of a pen. A paper is published, and you wake the next day to find that what you knew before you went to bed isn't so today. Yesterday's *Branhamella* is today's *Moraxella* – or was it the other way round?

The taxonomy of some bugs, however, is so established that re-classifying and renaming them would be unthinkable, and perhaps the best example of this is *Staphylococcus aureus*. Although doctors will abbreviate the name to *Staph aureus*, most likely you will know it under another name – golden staph. An aureus was a Roman gold coin and staphylococcus is from the Greek 'staphyle' (a bunch of grapes) and 'coccus' (granule). The Greco-Roman name beautifully describes the appearance of the bacteria in the laboratory – they really do look like a bunch of grapes under the microscope, and the colonies that grow on an agar plate are yellow.

I took very little notice of *Staph aureus* as a student and junior doctor. It was, to my mind, a pedestrian sort of bug. There was little romance associated with it – everybody had it on their skin, up their nose or in their groin. It caused tedious things like skin infections and abscesses and it had no international allure. Its main claim to fame was that some strains had developed a special characteristic that made them stand out in a crowd – resistance. The most famous strain is known mainly by its acronym – MRSA (Methicillin-resistant Staphylococcus aureus).

Antibiotic resistance is a fashionable subject in the early 21st century. Some authorities believe that we may be in the last decades of the 'Antibiotic Age', that soon the bacteria will win and we will be back to the 1930s, before the advent of sulphur drugs and penicillin. It is hard to pick up a medical journal without reading about the appearance of a germ that has mutated so that it is resistant to most antibiotics. There is no better way to frighten a patient than to inform them that they have an infection caused by a resistant organism. 'Oh my god, that's a superbug isn't it?' they usually say, and you can see family members trying to hide the fact that they have taken a small step back from the bedside. Often the patient's perception is that MRSA has flesh-eating capabilities and they will be banished to an isolation ward in the basement of the hospital, somewhere between the incinerator and the morgue. In reality MRSA is no more, and possibly less, dangerous than the common-or-garden variety *Staph aureus*. The so-called superbugs may be resistant to antibiotics but they are no more virulent than their antibiotic-sensitive cousins. Indeed, there is an evolutionary cost of developing resistance – the bacteria may actually become less pathogenic. The problem is that to treat the MRSA antibiotics have to be used that are less effective than the usual choices, have serious side-effects and toxicities, or are extremely expensive. For example, the drug linezolid which is sometimes used to treat MRSA costs around $120 a tablet, and a patient needs two tablets a day for a minimum of a week for the simplest infection, and much longer in the case of complicated infections.

MRSA is usually transmitted from patient to patient in hospital, mainly on the hands of the doctors and nurses who care for them. In our hospital, which has quite low rates of resistant organisms, we isolate all patients who are known to have MRSA to minimise its spread, This can have a negative psychological effect on some people, as they often feel stigmatised (conversely, others enjoy the quiet and relative privacy of the single room that their 'unclean' status confers). Some hospitals have so much MRSA that they are unable to offer enough single rooms, and so the patients are not segregated. Without antibiotic treatment most people with MRSA will naturally become clear of the bacteria over time, but this can take many months or even years.

While I am never happy when I learn that a patient has had an MRSA isolated from some part of their body, I only really get worried when it has grown in a specimen that was taken from a site in the body that should be sterile – say, an artificial joint or, worse, from their bloodstream. But if growing MRSA from the blood of a hospitalised patient is bad, I am even more disturbed when I learn of a patient who has not been in hospital and who has grown a *Staph aureus* in their blood which *is* sensitive to the routine antibiotics. Most doctors who are not specialists in infectious diseases don't get too fussed about this, but it is one of the most serious diagnoses that I can make.

More urgency in emergency

Medical systems around the world respond to certain problems in a stereotyped way. The reason that someone with chest pain triggers an immediate response in an emergency department is that a heart attack can kill you quickly and early intervention reduces the risk of death and subsequent complications.

In the 1970s if you survived a heart attack long enough to get to hospital the chance of leaving alive was about 80 per cent, and in the 1980s around 85 per cent. Today the chance of you making it home is about 93 per cent. One of the reasons for the continuing decline in the mortality rate from heart attacks in people admitted to hospital has been the rapidity of the medical response. The quality of a cardiology or emergency department can be gauged by the time it takes to get from the door of the hospital to the catheter laboratory where the patient's blocked artery can be opened up. A hospital's reputation can hinge on how quickly it achieves this, and it would be impossible for a doctor not to see a heart attack as an emergency requiring an immediate response.

Unfortunately, the response of most hospital systems to patients presenting with infections, even the most obvious and serious types, is much more relaxed. A patient who has grown *Staph aureus* in his blood is said to have bacteraemia or, more colloquially, blood poisoning. The bug can get into the bloodstream through small breaches in the skin caused by simple cuts and scratches, via things inserted for medical reasons – an intravenous cannula, for example – and from needles used to inject illicit drugs. A patient with *Staph aureus* bacteraemia will initially feel unwell, may develop a headache, muscle and back pains, and experience chills and rigours (shivering fits). If the disease progresses the infected person's blood pressure drops, they become delirious and eventually slip into a coma.

The severity of the disease varies enormously from patient to patient, depending on age, general state of health and, it would seem, providence. Although it is no surprise that an elderly patient with heart disease and diabetes will do very poorly if they get a *Staph aureus* infection, I have seen fit young people with the same infection become sick in the morning, be in intensive care that night and dead by the end of the week. It would be reasonable to assume that the earlier a patient with *Staph aureus* in their blood receives antibiotics the better their chance of survival. At the Canberra Hospital we have been collecting data on patients with infections in their blood for over ten years, and the information provides a unique insight into what happens to patients with these infections in Australia. The study has shown that a patient who develops *Staph aureus* bacteraemia has about a 25 per cent chance of being dead within six months (the percentage is higher in many countries) regardless of how healthy or old they are when they get the infection. In other words, if you go into hospital with *Staph aureus* in your blood you are between three and four times more likely to be dead within the year than if you had arrived with a heart attack. This is a fact little known to doctors – or their patients – and few hospitals have the same protocols in place for the rapid identification and treatment of bloodstream infections as they do for heart attacks. Few, if any, hospitals could tell you how long it takes a patient with bacteraemia to receive antibiotics.

Recently two of my students calculated the time it took for patients in our hospital with suspected meningitis, another condition where every second counts, to receive antibiotics. The median time of just over three hours was consistent with results from overseas hospitals, but it highlights the different approach that medical staff take when it comes to infections compared to affairs of the heart.

Why do intelligent and motivated people act so differently when the results of delay can be so devastating? Perhaps it is the immediacy of the consequences of a heart attack that prompt medical staff into action – the patient's heart can stop without a second's warning, the muscle of the heart can be damaged so badly that it can't pump enough blood around the body and the effect – a breathless, gasping patient – is right in front of the doctor's eyes.

Every week we diagnose at least one new staph bloodstream infection in our hospital. I know that the earlier we diagnose the infection, the better the patient's chances of a full recovery, but I also know that a proportion of patients will not receive the right antibiotic, given at the right dose, for the right duration. As a result, this invisible little bunch of grapes will have seeded itself in occult parts of the human body that it invaded and reappear in a few days or weeks. This time it will demand treatment by dint of its severe manifestations – a heart valve may be infected, an abscess may have formed in the spine or a muscle, or in the brain. Those of us who treat these complications appreciate what the absence of an urgent initial response can lead to, but we have failed in the main to convey this sense of urgency to our colleagues who have the opportunity to initiate treatment.

Most serious bloodstream infections start in the community – well before the patient has been anywhere near a hospital – and there is not a lot that we can do to prevent them occurring in the first place. Sometimes, however, the infection *is* the fault of the medical system, and the consequences can be a grizzly showcase for its failings.

'Just don't mention this in front of his mother'

He was admitted to the hospital after a fight outside a nightclub. He had been punched in the face by a drunk who was aiming at someone else. The blow had fractured the man's cheekbone, and his face had been badly cut when he fell on broken glass in the gutter. After the ambulance arrived a paramedic inserted an intravenous cannula in his left arm, just at the elbow. When he got to the hospital a surgeon assessed that he needed a procedure to push his jaw back into place, but there was no theatre time available that night, or the next day, and it was 48 hours before he had his operation. He recovered well after the surgery but on the third day after admission developed a high temperature. He was seen by a series of residents over three shifts. They examined his face, chest and wounds, took blood tests and requested a chest X-ray, but didn't order any antibiotics. His temperature fluctuated, and while he felt reasonable for most of the day, when it went up he looked and felt dreadful. On the fourth day he developed rigours and a set of blood cultures was taken. The next day, a Saturday, he was much sicker, and his girlfriend said she thought he was not making any sense. The laboratory rang the ward to say the blood cultures were positive for *Staph aureus*. The medical registrar was called, but it was an hour before he could see the patient. When he arrived he was appalled by what he saw: from the end of the bed it was apparent to him that the patient had developed septic shock. He made an emergency call, and soon the room was full of doctors, nurses and orderlies.

'He needs to move to the intensive care immediately', the registrar said. Toxins from the multiplying bacteria had entered the patient's circulation and initiated a cascade of events. His heart rate had risen but his blood pressure had fallen, consequently the heart was unable to pump enough blood to provide adequate oxygen to all the tissues. The body's automatic response was to regulate the flow of blood, supplying the most important organs – the brain and heart –at the expense of the kidneys, liver and the gut. These can only continue to function with a reduced blood flow for a short time before they start to fail – the kidneys first, then the lungs and finally the brain. The patient was confused and delirious, then his consciousness faded –a sequence of events very difficult to reverse.

On the ward he was given intravenous fluid to try to increase his blood pressure. Additional oxygen was also administered, but it was clear his blood oxygen level was still falling. A tube was inserted into his trachea, but his lungs were waterlogged and stiff from fluid that had escaped from capillaries leaking because of the bacteria in his blood. His blood pressure remained dangerously low and he needed to be transferred to the ICU urgently so that he could receive the adrenaline-like drugs that could bring it up to a safer level. The bedside was cluttered with people busy with lines and tubes and monitors. His mother stood outside the room, silent, ashen, trying to hold onto her composure as she felt it running away from her. The ICU registrar was there now.

'Everyone needs to hurry up a bit and get this move underway please', she said as she walked around the bed while the medical registrar filled her in on the details. She was listening and examining the patient at the same time. Suddenly, she interrupted her colleague in mid-sentence.

'What is this?' she asked, pointing to the intravenous cannula in the patient's left arm, at the elbow. 'How long has this been in?' She looked more closely. The cannula site was red, and as she touched the surrounding skin a drop of yellow pus welled up at the edges of the plastic tube. The medical registrar didn't know when the cannula was inserted: there was nothing written on the dressing around the cannula and no documentation in the medical notes. The only reference to when it was put in came from the ambulance officer's notes from five days before.

The ICU registrar pulled out the cannula and handed it to the nurse, telling him to send the tip of the cannula to the laboratory for culture. This was a formality: the *Staph aureus* almost certainly entered the man's bloodstream soon after the assault, through the breach in the skin caused by inserting the cannula. As the days passed the number of bugs multiplied exponentially, so that by the time the ICU registrar spotted the cannula the bacteria were well established in the man's circulation. The patient was wheeled out of the ward, his bed now a moving ICU, packed with monitors, infusion machines, oxygen bottles and suspended fluids. The medical registrar stayed in the ward. The ICU staff were in control now.

A medical student, who had been watching the events play out from a corner of the room, asked him how this could have happened.

'That cannula should have been removed as soon as he arrived in the emergency department and a new one put in', the registrar said. 'The new one should have come out within 48 hours, 72 hours max.'

'The hospital should have a policy about this', said the student.

'It does – I've just told you the policy', the registrar replied, shrugging his shoulders.

'But why don't people follow the policy if there is one?' asked the student.

'You tell me', said the registrar, walking out of the room. 'Just don't mention any of this in front of his mother, will you.'

The patient died later that night – his lungs were so damaged that it was impossible to get enough oxygen into them. His heart stopped and could not be restarted.

He was 24 years old.

Time for a little respect

We could use the tragedy that I have described to pick apart any number of systemic failings, but my main point is to illustrate the potency of a common bacterium. Resistance to antibiotics is an important subject for discussion, but it can be a little distracting. Staphylococcal infections kill hundreds of Australians each year and put thousands in hospital, yet the vast majority of the responsible strains are sensitive to cheap and safe antibiotics. There is no vaccine available for *Staph aureus* and there is nothing on the horizon.

The generation who grew up in the pre-antibiotic age knew very well the capacity of bland bacteria to cause terrible sickness. But today respect for the power of bacteria sometimes seems to be limited to those who see the late manifestations of infections. In hospital practice, working at the bottom of a 'diagnostic sieve' that funnels the sickest our way, my fellow 'infectionistas' and I have frequent opportunities to see the uncommon life-threatening consequences of bacterial invasion. Perhaps we are too nice, maybe we lack the swagger and metaphorical cojones of the cardiologists, because we are unable to get many of our colleagues to recognise that an infection in the blood is a slow-motion heart attack – less dramatic when played at normal speed, but just as deadly in fast-forward.

8

Severe *and* acute?
That has to be bad!

SARS coronavirus (SARS-CoV) – a positive-stranded RNA virus
first discovered in 2003 when it triggered a near pandemic of a
previously unknown disease, causing a high rate of pneumonia
and respiratory failure among the people infected and the death
of 8 per cent of them. The virus is thought to have originated
in the cat-like civet in China and moved into the human
population because of a growing local appetite for exotic meats.
Within weeks of the initial outbreak the disease had spread to
nearly 40 countries.

'His flight was madness: when our actions do not, our fears
make us traitors.' (from *Macbeth*, by William Shakespeare,
1564–1616)

During the early days of the SARS (severe acute respiratory syndrome) epidemic in 2003 I received an email from a colleague, D.,
an infectious diseases physician working in Singapore. He posted
the message in the online forum that the society representing the
speciality uses to canvass opinion and seek advice about difficult
clinical problems. I had worked with D. in Darwin for several
years. He had a dry, even mordant, sense of humour and was

never one for hyperbole. During the Timor refugee crisis in 1999 he had remained a calm and solid presence, admitting patients to hospital in Darwin as the need arose, never over-reacting, always helpful but never seeking any praise for his actions. He enjoyed the good life and rolled with the punches that are an unavoidable part of medical practice. He was laid-back – which sometimes disguised his insight – and he could always be relied on to bring us down to earth when we started to get too excited about things.

The stories that were appearing in the press about SARS were very concerning, and when things are moving as quickly as they were in those first days and weeks, the news media was the fastest way to get information. When I saw D's name at the top of the email I knew that I was going to get a sober and balanced view of what was going on in his part of the world. It would be good to take a deep breath and realise that the growing hysteria was misplaced and that SARS, as many of us suspected, was a bit of a beat-up. The fact that the WHO had released the first Global Alert in its history should have already made me a bit more concerned than I was, but as I read D's email I started to get a bit worried.

He talked about the deaths from SARS of hospital staff in Singapore – all young and previously fit people. He said that he was taking his own temperature several times a day and had decided that if he developed a fever he would move into his office at the hospital and not go home for fear of transmitting the illness to his wife and young family. His tone was not in any way shrill, but he was obviously quite fearful of the possibility of contagion. If D. was writing like this, then SARS must be the 'real deal'. And if I harboured any residual doubts about its seriousness, these were finally dispelled in late March, when the Rolling Stones cancelled their upcoming Hong Kong concerts – if Keith Richards was frightened of something, then so was I.

The future had arrived: for years we had been anticipating that a highly contagious pandemic influenza strain with a high

problem with him being a little apprehensive – it is a normal response and sharpens your ability to protect yourself. 'Come on and I'll show you how to gown and mask.'

But it was clear that he wasn't going to follow me. In fact as I spoke he was heading down the corridor and out of the ward. I was stunned by his behaviour but didn't follow him. I had other priorities for the time being, so I let him go. This was the first time I had ever seen a doctor refuse point-blank to see a patient because of a personal fear of contagion, but I had to acknowledge his honesty, and as I walked down the corridor I realised that I didn't really want to do this either. But if I was going to ask the residents and the nurses to care for the patient, then I had to be prepared to see her as well. I carefully put on the duckbill N95 mask that forms a seal around your face and filters out viruses and bacteria. I put on the goggles – which fogged-up immediately – and the disposable protective gown. Then, taking a deep breath in the hallway, I opened the door to the isolation room and walked inside.

An hour later, after examining her and assessing her risk of exposure after she told me about her travel movements, I had concluded that she probably didn't have SARS – it was much more likely that she had what is known as an atypical pneumonia. But we would run the tests just the same and keep her in isolation until we had an all-clear from the laboratory. I spoke to the chief health officer that night and he pointed out that because 11 days had elapsed between her possible exposure and the onset of symptoms, she did not meet the WHO case-definition for SARS. He was correct, of course, but it was right to err on the side of caution in those early, uncertain days of the epidemic.

Transmission time is the Achilles heel

At the peak of the epidemic, which coincided with the first days of the second Gulf war, my wife and I left for a conference in Paris. As we checked in at the airport we discovered, to our considerable delight, that we had been upgraded, not to business but to first class. The reason for this unexpected largesse became apparent when we boarded – there was hardly anyone on the plane. Our stopover at Changi airport was like walking through a post-armageddon science fiction movie set. The halls were nearly empty and all the attendants were wearing face masks. We had our masks in our pockets, but we reasoned that because there was so much distance between everyone we wouldn't need to wear them. The real reason, however, was that I felt a little silly putting on a mask in these circumstances. I would, it turns out, rather be exposed to a deadly virus than to the risk of embarrassment.

We, and all but 774 inhabitants of the earth survived SARS, which, to the relief and even surprise of the medical community, disappeared as quickly as it arrived. The causative agent was identified with remarkable speed: within months a previously unknown member of the coronavirus virus family was isolated and its genetic code elucidated. But it would be simple observations of the way the virus behaved in the humans it infected (that is, its epidemiology) that would provide the best insight into why it was so easily contained.

The fundamental difference between SARS and influenza was the time it took for infected patients to start excreting the virus. This is different from the incubation period, which is the time between exposure to infection and development of symptoms. It is a little known distinction. People with SARS did not reach the peak of contagiousness until they had been ill for nearly ten days. This meant that quarantining sufferers as quickly as possible had a powerful effect on reducing transmission to others.

Most viruses are spread before those carrying them feel sick, or when they are in the earliest phases of the illness. Quarantining people with measles, for example, is of limited value because they have been excreting the virus in their respiratory secretions (coughs, sneezes, and so on) for several days before the typical rash develops. Similarly, people with influenza are highly infectious almost the moment they become ill and it is practically impossible to quarantine people quickly enough to completely interrupt transmission.

The rise and fall of SARS is a beautiful demonstration of evolution in action. The disease emerged for two reasons: a change in the particular coronavirus (a mutation which made the virus more virulent and easier to transmit to and between humans); and a change in the way humans interact with the environment (a growing appetite for exotic meat in China that saw the virus spread from civet cats and possibly other wildlife to humans). There was little or no pre-existing immunity in the population, so the disease spread quickly and killed around 8 per cent of those infected. But the Achilles heel of the virus was the time it took for those infected to become infectious. It is likely that hundreds of similar episodes of emergence and then disappearance of infectious agents have occurred throughout human history – it is only the fittest organisms that survive and establish themselves as human diseases. Eventually the illnesses caused by the surviving pathogens can only be controlled through vaccination or environmental changes such as sanitation and better housing.

No one in the medical communities where SARS occurred was left untouched by tragedy: my Singapore-born registrar in Canberra lost two friends during the epidemic. SARS reminded the health professions that their work is intrinsically fraught with danger. The emergence of HIV in the 1980s had done this for a previous generation, but the lessons had receded into memory. A major difference too was that the risk to medical staff from HIV was extremely low, while the likelihood of SARS transmission was substantial. SARS showed that if the medical profession was threatened, infection control became a priority, not just a set of annoying rules often interpreted as being designed to slow work-flows and make life more complicated.

I suppose I should have anticipated that doctors and nurses would respond more to a threat to themselves than to the altru-istic motivator of the prevention and reduction of infections in their patients. Infection control, like immunisation, can be a victim of its own success. When it is working well, good infec-tion control practice prevents disease and avoids prolonged and unexpected hospital stays. The person who didn't get an infection after their operation never phones to thank you. The nurse who didn't stab herself on the needle in the linen bag has no reason to be grateful for your policy. The people involved in infection control around the world spend their professional lives being more disappointed than surprised. They are always looking for incentives that will change people's behaviour, but experience tells them that a virtue-based approach will not work: 'doing the right thing' is so very 20th century. Many of the failures of modern medical systems are due to a lack of imagination or, to use another word, empathy. We appear to lack the ability to *imagine* ourselves in the place of another and have to wait until we are actually *in* the other's shoes before a risk becomes authentic. SARS was seen as a dress rehearsal for the international response to a virulent pandemic influenza strain and it highlighted the best and worst of the medical system and its people. But most important of all, SARS made infection control real for medical people – something that it seems every new generation can only learn for itself.

9

The pox under our noses

Herpes simplex virus type 2 (HSV-2) – a member of the
Herpesviridae family and the commonest cause of genital herpes.
There are eight human herpes viruses and all but HSV-2 cause
common childhood infections, including its closest relative, HSV-
1, the bringer of cold sores. Although the illnesses that they cause
are usually short-lived, herpes viruses evade the immune system
and establish life-long latent infection in their human hosts.
However, the vast majority of those infected are never aware that
they carry these viruses.

'Oh how can I forget you when there is always something there to
remind me?' (from 'Always something there to remind me', lyrics
by Burt Bacharach, 1928–)

It is a rare man who enjoys pulling down his pants for a doctor.
They exist, but their diagnosis is usually psychiatric rather than
venereological. For everyone else, even the sudden discovery
of something nasty on one's genitalia does not over-ride the
anticipatory embarrassment of having to show it to someone
in a clinic. One of the lines that we use to reassure our more
anxious patients in this setting is, 'Don't worry, there's nothing I
haven't seen before'. The line probably goes some way to easing
the transition from clothed to fully exposed, and I learnt to use

it early in my career.

One morning many years ago I collected a young man who, the receptionist warned me, had been pacing around the waiting room. He walked down the hall with a wide-based, legs-apart gait that was the only thing that made him look like John Wayne – everything else about him said Ricky Gervais. I took his history and learnt that a week previously he had had a brief but torrid sexual affair with a Norwegian backpacker whom he had met in a bar. Five days after she had left town in the back of a Combi van he had developed a headache, muscle aches and felt 'off'. He attributed his illness to flu, but the following day he woke with tingling and discomfort along the shaft of his penis. By the next day his whole member was red, swollen, and exquisitely painful.

'Well', I said, motioning him towards the examination couch. 'We'd better have a look'. The resolve that had brought him to the clinic suddenly evaporated and he didn't move from his chair.

'Don't worry', I continued. 'There's nothing I haven't seen before. Come on jump up on the couch.'

He pulled down his trousers and underpants to reveal a swollen penis, ulcerated along its length and sticky with a yellowish secretion. But most memorably, the penis was bent in two parts, the first 90-degree bend close to the base, the second, also at 90 degrees, a few centimetres further along and in the other direction. The expression on my face must have changed because he looked at me with the eyes of a labrador puppy.

'What's the matter?' he intoned.

'It's hard to say.'

'What do you mean?'

'Well, it's like nothing I've ever seen before.'

I called in one of my colleagues, a male nurse with years of sexual-health experience. I asked him what he thought.

'I think this is a case of Bill Clinton penis', he said with a perfectly straight face after inspecting the evidence in front of him. The young man on the couch looked at me in a way that indicated that he questioned the sanity of my nursing assistant. I was of the same mind, until it suddenly clicked. The diagnosis was a condition colloquially called saxophone penis and the Monica Lewinsky scandal engulfing the US presidency at the time had given rise to a joke about Bill Clinton's manhood and his preferred musical instrument.

'Tell me what this means?' implored our patient.

I told him that he had herpes.

Off the toilet wall and on to the news-stand

The front-cover story of *Time* magazine in August 1982 was devoted to an incurable sexually transmitted virus. The article described how the comrades at the barricades of the sexual revolution were reaping the rewards of their nocturnal labours of the preceding two decades – and the name of the prize was not AIDS but genital herpes (a report about AIDS would provide the front cover material just six months later). For a subterranean infection like herpes to breach the surface of polite middle-class society, the disease must have reached a level in the community unseen since the syphilis epidemic that affected the GIs returning from the Second World War. The problem was that, in contrast to the 'traditional' venereal diseases, gonorrhoea and syphilis, which were treatable with antibiotics, there was then no treatment for genital herpes.

The graffiti in the toilets of my medical school at the time of the magazine article asked 'What is the difference between true love and herpes?' The answer was 'herpes lasts for ever'. 'How does herpes leave hospitals?' enquired another anonymous wit. 'On crutches'. Of course. I occasionally learnt things in the lecture theatres as well: herpes is from the Latin 'to creep', and I discovered that there are eight human herpes viruses. Also, that there are two animal herpes viruses that on rare occasions cause human disease – the herpes B virus, which occurs in macaque monkeys and has been transferred mainly to laboratory workers, and the mouse herpes virus. Collectively, the herpes viruses are the Howard Hugheses of the viral kingdom: they like to keep a low profile and they have some strange habits. The evolutionary strategy that they have adopted is to cause mild, if troublesome, infection in childhood and to then remain dormant for the rest of their host's life by hiding somewhere in the body, usually in the nervous system or in the bone marrow. Periodically, some of them reactivate for short periods, when they can be transmitted to a new human host, reproduce, and thus perpetuate their existence. Herpes viruses rarely cause death, but infection occurring later in life or soon after birth can be very severe.

Best caught young

The herpes virus that causes chicken pox and shingles is known as the varicella zoster virus or VZV. Chicken pox is also known as varicella, the diminutive form of variola, the Latin for smallpox. Shingles, also known as zoster (from the Greek for 'belt' because of its characteristic appearance on the skin when it affects the trunk) occurs when the virus reactivates later in life.

Chicken pox is the least dangerous of the classic childhood illnesses. Unlike measles – which can cause pneumonia and encephalitis, and even kill younger children – chicken pox was almost a good disease to have: you didn't have to go to school and apart from the itchy scabs and the embarrassing pink of the calamine lotion, you could enjoy your week of quarantine with comics and day-time television. Death and serious neurological complications occurred, but they were extremely rare, and dwarfed by the number of complications caused by other childhood illnesses, such as scarlet fever and whooping cough.

Chicken pox in an adult, on the other hand, is an unpleasant and serious disease. Smokers who develop the infection are especially at risk of life-threatening pneumonia. I have treated several smokers who have needed admission to the intensive care unit, their lungs full of chicken pox blisters which stop the usual flow of oxygen from the atmosphere to their bloodstream. Pregnant women are also at increased risk of complicated disease, and this can be a disaster for them and for their unborn child.

After childhood infection, VZV lies dormant in the nerve cells. Shingles occurs when the virus re-activates in adulthood, but instead of producing chicken pox it now causes painful blistering along the path of sensory nerves. Shingles can affect any part of the body, but the trunk, arms and face are the most frequently affected parts. The disease becomes more common in late middle age and at least half the population can expect to suffer an attack in their lifetime. If it occurs in younger people, an underlying cause of immune suppression should always be considered (in Africa and other high-prevalence countries, shingles in a young person is a common indicator of HIV infection). Some unfortunate people develop a terrible, persisting syndrome called post-herpetic neuralgia, which can be debilitating because of prolonged episodes of severe pain along the path of the nerves that were originally involved. It can be extremely difficult to treat successfully.

Chicken pox will soon be as little known to the coming generation of parents as diphtheria and tetanus were to mine. All children in the developed world are now being offered routine immunisation against the disease, and, as the vaccine program is rolled out, even children who haven't been vaccinated will be protected by herd immunity *(see page 68)*. These unvaccinated individuals will, however, be susceptible to chicken pox if they travel to countries without vaccine programs or are exposed to the large pool of adults with shingles. Vaccine-related immunity may wane with time and it is quite possible that the vaccine will lead to more adult chicken pox, with all its attendant complications, unless the uptake of the vaccine in children is high and boosters are available in adult life for those who have lost their immunity. A vaccine for shingles is now licensed in Australia, but it has not yet found a place in routine care.

Something going around

Glandular fever, another well known disease of young people, is caused by the Epstein Barr virus (EBV), also a member of the herpes family. Cytomegalovirus or CMV, a disease associated with HIV and other causes of immunosuppression, is another scion (*see page 33*).

Up to 90 per cent of the population will catch EBV in childhood and develop a brief illness which makes the child a bit grizzly and feverish for a few days. Their GP quite rightly, if a little non-specifically, will diagnose a 'virus that's going around', and it is rare to investigate or definitively diagnose the infection at this stage. By adolescence, the majority of young people will have been exposed to EBV, but the minority who haven't are at risk of developing glandular fever that, by longstanding convention, waits until the day before an important exam to strike. This disease, characterised by sore throat, swollen glands, high temperatures and extreme tiredness, is known to parents and feared by teenagers, but is a much less common manifestation of EBV infection than that rarely diagnosed, mild infection of childhood described above. The post-glandular fever syndrome of 'chronic fatigue' is also much rarer than is commonly held and true reactivation of the illness is rarer still. Unfortunately hundreds of young people receive an erroneous diagnosis of chronic glandular fever every year. In adulthood, EBV infection can be a diagnostic dilemma – here the disease rarely causes the 'typical' glandular fever symptoms, and a combination of high fevers, malaise and blood test abnormalities may be the only symptoms.

The rare patient in their 60s or 70s who has managed to escape EBV infection until then may spend weeks or months being investigated for the cause of their fever before a simple antibody test reveals the answer.

The most recently discovered of the eight herpes viruses affecting humans are rather unimaginatively called human herpes viruses 6, 7 and 8 (HHV-6, HHV-7 and HHV-8). The first two cause the mild childhood rash called roseola, which just about every child will catch, and they never produce any serious complications. HHV-8, however, is the cause of Kaposi's sarcoma, an otherwise extremely rare cancer of the blood vessels which became a common manifestation of AIDS during the early years of the HIV epidemic (*see page 33*).

It started with a kiss

The next two herpes viruses affecting humans, herpes simplex type 1 (HSV-1) and herpes simplex type 2 (HSV-2) are the respective causes of cold sores and genital herpes. It is an acronym that has caused me great amusement since Holden badged a high-performance range of vehicles with the letters HSV. When I have pulled up to one of them at traffic lights I have often been tempted to lower a window and say to the, usually mulleted, driver: 'You do know what HSV *really* stands for, don't you mate?' Self-preservation instincts have prevailed, however.

Cold sores are the blistery bane of the skier and the nervous debutante. Like VZV, HSV hides in the peripheral nerves and can be reactivated by stress, illness, immune suppression, the menstrual cycle and bad luck, among other things. Unlike shingles, which is usually a solitary if memorable event for the sufferer, HSV can recur frequently and at the most inopportune moment. I remember pointing out to friends what looked like cold sores on Judy Davis's lips in the 1979 film *My Brilliant Career*. One of them was a whopper, and what problems they must have caused the make-up lady and the director: the evolving changes in the cold sores would have made shooting out of sequence a nightmare. It was one of my first presumptive cinematic diagnoses, but I have never been able to confirm it virologically, alas.

Most adults are infected with HSV-1 but only a small proportion suffers cold sores. It is unclear why some people get them and others don't, but most who catch the infection do so by coming in contact with someone who doesn't even know they are infected – we call these people asymptomatic excretors. The usually superfluous advice to avoid kissing people with big herpes on their lips is driven more by aesthetic considerations than by infection control – most people will pick up their cold sores from an asymptomatic excretor. It is an unfortunate fact that every kiss is a game of microbiological Russian roulette – you never know which lips are loaded.

And so to the herpes virus that my male patient at the start of this chapter had – genital herpes (HSV-2). One in eight Australians has antibodies to HSV-2, (16 per cent of women and 8 per cent of men), but as in the case of the cold sore herpes only around 20 per cent of these people will ever know that they are infected: symptomatic disease is only the, err, tip of the herpes iceberg. But if you do develop symptoms you can be quite unwell. HSV-2 sufferers can experience a severe flu-like illness for a few days and then develop a painful eruption of herpes blisters on the genitals. I have on occasion had to admit young women with a primary genital herpes attack to hospital for pain relief, and sometimes a urinary catheter has had to be inserted so that they can pass urine. However, the fear of a diagnosis of genital herpes is sometimes more distressing than the disease itself; the vast majority of people with genital herpes infection have much milder symptoms, and while attacks can recur for many years, or even for life in some cases, the relapses usually become less frequent and less severe.

For the majority of sufferers, once they get past the hype and the anxiety of the unknown, the infection is just a damned nuisance – essentially a cold sore on your penis or vulva, and much easier to cover up than a cold sore. Having said that, the psychosexual consequences of a diagnosis of HSV-2 can be devastating for some people and careful counselling of everyone who is diagnosed with the condition is essential.

Infection with a herpes simplex virus is like a Jesuit primary school education – once you have had it, it has you for life. The ability of herpes infections to come back again and again over a lifetime consolidates their good Catholic qualities – the consequences of a deed perpetrated in the distant past can impose themselves upon your reconstructed present.

An interesting change in the epidemiology of the disease has occurred in the past ten years. Infection with HSV-1 appears to provide modest protection from HSV-2 infection. The bigger your family and the poorer your socio-economic circumstances, the more likely you are to have contracted HSV-1 in childhood. Paradoxically, rising affluence and the trend towards smaller families in the last 40 years means the chance of children picking up the cold sore virus has decreased, and it is plausible that the rise of sexually acquired HSV-2 is due, at least in part, to the declining numbers of people carrying the HSV-1 virus. The other intriguing change has been the rise in the number of cases of genital herpes that are caused by the cold sore virus: an increasing proportion of people who are diagnosed with genital herpes are found to have HSV-1, not HSV-2. Again, this is not entirely explicable, but it may be due to the vogue for oral sex among members of Generation Y, something which may be associated with their well known predilection for doing two things at once – texting while they drive is another example.

HSV-1 and HSV-2 infections are very difficult to prevent – there is no vaccine on the market and little prospect of one in the next 15 years. Condoms, which provide excellent protection against HIV, gonorrhoea and chlamydia, don't work so well for herpes because the latex can't cover all the areas that are potentially excreting the virus or exposed to its transmission. It's like taking a shower with a raincoat on: parts of you still get wet.

Treatment has been available for 25 years and is now relatively cheap (the original drug is off-patent), but it's a herpes – the virus isn't eradicated, just suppressed. The pharmaceutical companies love herpes because it is incurable and common, and they compete for market share for the two drugs that are still in patent. It seems that all that blisters *is* gold, for some.

A lot is made of the value of antiviral treatment for recurrences of genital herpes, but in reality the benefits are marginal. However, the drugs are safe and there is little harm in taking a drug that has a small but definite chance of either aborting a recurrence (if it is taken in the earliest stages) or shortening the duration of symptoms. Nevertheless, you have to treat 20 patients to abort one recurrence, and while the duration of a recurrence drops from six days to four days, the last two days of a recurrent attack are usually quite mild anyway. Treatment of a first attack is much more effective – the duration of symptoms is reduced from an average of 21 days to about ten days. The same applies for HSV-1 – there is considerable benefit in treating primary attacks but less for recurrences of the disease. Topical antiviral ointments and creams have very limited effect on the course of primary or recurrent infections by either virus.

Some HSV-2 patients with really debilitating disease caused by multiple recurrences are treated with chronic suppressive treatment, which means taking one or two tablets a day for as long as they want to stay free of symptoms. For young people who haven't reached an age when blood pressure and cholesterol pills have become a part of the daily routine, the idea of taking medication in this way is not always acceptable.

Having played down the severity of illness in most groups of people, there is an important exception – that of the newborn baby. A woman who experiences a primary attack of genital herpes in late pregnancy has a substantial risk of transmitting the infection to her child during labour, and this can be fatal for the child unless treatment is started immediately after birth. Fortunately, a primary attack in this setting is very rare. The much more common problem of reactivation of previously acquired genital herpes in late pregnancy carries only a small risk for the baby of infection at birth, but it is important to know if lesions are present at the time of delivery and to avoid a vaginal birth if possible. However, to reduce the need for a caesarian section, some authorities now recommend antiviral treatment in late pregnancy for women who are known to suffer multiple recurrent attacks of HSV-2

The swabs from my patient with saxophone penis came back positive for HSV-2 and I had already started him on an antiviral drug. It was a much less apprehensive young man who returned to the clinic the following week. The inflammation of the skin caused by the herpes, which had resulted in swelling of the underlying penile tissue and had bent the shaft into its characteristic conformation, had now settled. Without any prompting he pulled down his pants and jumped up on the couch to show me that his anatomy had returned to normal. We talked for some time about condoms and safe sex and the chance of recurrent attacks of herpes, but his mind was elsewhere. Norway, I think.

10

Cultures that stink

Bacteroides fragilis – a multi-shaped Gram-negative bacterium
that lives in the human gut. One of dozens of bacterial species
that do not require oxygen to multiply, *B. fragilis* is a common
cause of severe infections that complicate abdominal conditions
such as appendicitis, diverticulitis and bowel obstruction.
Anaerobic bacteria produce infections that have a distinctive and
extremely unpleasant smell.

'The past is the only dead thing that smells sweet.' (from 'Early
One Morning', by Edward Thomas, 1878–1917)

It is sometimes possible to make a diagnosis just by using your
sense of smell. It doesn't happen very often in this age of medicine that is so dominated by laboratory and radiological investigations. Clinical examination is, for many doctors, a neglected
art and even, in the opinion of some, a waste of time. But nothing
beats the satisfaction that you get when you work out what is
going on by the simple method of listening, looking, touching
and smelling. (Tasting, I am pleased to say, is no longer part of
the medical school curriculum.)

The young patient who is hyperventilating, confused and
dehydrated and whose breath smells of nail polish remover
probably has diabetic ketoacidosis. Because of a lack of insulin,

the body is unable to utilise the sugars in the blood that provide energy for the cells. To get energy in this circumstance, the body has to break down fats, and the by-products of this process are called ketone bodies. When they appear in the blood in excess, ketone bodies are broken down to form acetone – the main component of nail polish remover – which produces the characteristic sweet, pungent smell of the sick diabetic. You can smell acetone on the breath of many patients who don't have diabetes – anyone who is fasting can become ketotic. Indeed, forcing the body to break down fat by limiting the intake of carbohydrates (sugar) is the stated intention of the famous Atkin's diet, which, if you have tried it yourself or have friends who have embarked on it, you will know can be quite depressing. Indeed, and with apologies to Thoreau, it has been said that on this diet massive men lead lives of quiet fat-respiration.

A rose by any other name

There are other olfactory diagnoses that are very easy to make. One of the complications of a peptic ulcer of the stomach or duodenum is bleeding. The ulcer can erode an artery, and when the arterial blood leaks into the lumen of the bowel and mixes with the hydrochloric acid of the stomach it undergoes a chemical alteration, and its colour changes from red to black. By the time it reaches the large intestine, the ulcer sufferer's stool takes on a 'tarry' appearance from this blood. These black faeces are called melaena (from the Greek word melanos, for black). I cannot convey the power of the effect that the odour of melaena has on you the first time you smell it – you really have to be there. And once you have been there you probably won't want to go there ever again. One person's melaena is another's freshly cut hay, however; I trained under a gastroenterologist who would stride into the gastro ward each morning, take a few exaggerated deep breaths and, in a homage to the character played by Robert Duvall on the beach in the film *Apocalypse Now*, proclaim his love for the smell of melaena in the morning.

Some smells are a little more subtle. When the liver of a patient with cirrhosis has been damaged so badly that all that is left is scar tissue, the organ is unable to break down a particular amino acid which circulates in the blood. The build-up of this toxin results in a sweet musty smell on the breath known by the medical name of foetor hepaticus. You have to get quite close up to your patient to detect it, but being alert to it allows the attentive doctor to recognise that the patient is on the edge of an abyss and urgent treatment for the liver failure is required.

Many of my patients smoke – which I suppose is one of the reasons that they become my patients in the first place – but not all of them smell the same. Why does one patient who smokes 20 cigarettes a day take the reek of tobacco smoke with them when they leave my room, while another heavy smoker pumps out the stink of tobacco and, worse, leaves the odour lingering when they have left? I have to open the windows and blast the room with the air conditioner to make it a suitable space for the next patient. In one of my clinics where there is no window or control over the air conditioner, I sometimes resort to air freshener, which is usually disastrous because the hospital-grade fragrance is worse than the stale tobacco smoke smell it is supposed to cover up.

Some bacterial infections have characteristic smells. One of the main distinctions that microbiologists make between bacteria is whether or not they need oxygen to grow in the laboratory. The oxygen-requiring bacteria are called aerobes and those that don't need oxygen are called anaerobes. It will come as no surprise to many spouses that the gas that exists in the intestine is not oxygen and so most of the organisms that live there are anaerobes. They reside there happily for much of the time, causing no harm unless they escape from the confines of the bowel. As we age, many of us develop little out-pouchings of bowel, called diverticula. If one of these becomes blocked it can perforate and faeces spread into the peritoneal cavity – a place which is normally sterile. The patient develops a fever, abdominal pain, and can become very sick indeed if the bacteria enter the bloodstream. Usually an abscess forms and, since antibiotics can't penetrate into a collection of pus, the abscess must be drained, either by an operation or through a long needle guided with the aid of ultrasound or a CT scan. If the pus that is obtained is foul-smelling, the diagnosis of an anaerobic infection can be suspected well before the results from the microbiology laboratory are available. A compost heap can have this smell if it is not properly aerated for exactly the same reason – the dominance of the anaerobic bacteria over the less offensive smelling aerobics.

Anaerobic bacteria live in your mouth too, although they are usually different from the ones that inhabit the lower gut. In the oral cavity they conspire to produce, among other things, two especially unattractive results: bad breath and dental caries. Most of us don't consider tooth decay to be an infectious disease, but it most certainly is. Plaque, a substance of obsessive interest to the dentist but ignored by infectious diseases doctors, is a beautiful culture medium for anaerobes, and its physical removal is crucial for the prevention of cavity formation. Plaque creates a barrier to oxygen, allowing the anaerobes to flourish and produce acidic waste products that attack the tooth enamel. If things really get out of hand, the anaerobes can produce a severe gingivitis called Vincent's angina or, as it became known during the First World War, trench mouth (a condition from which Marilyn Monroe is said to have suffered after having her wisdom teeth extracted). As they consume the nutrients provided by the plaque, the bacteria also produce a selection of aromatic amines (ammonia compounds) that cause halitosis. The back of the tongue can also harbour anaerobes, which act as a backup source of these halitosis-producing substances.

If we travel south a metre or so, we may encounter the commonest cause of vaginal discharge – bacterial vaginosis. Usually referred to by its initials BV, this unpleasant problem is characterised by a population explosion of anaerobic bacteria in the vagina coupled with a paucity of the 'good' bacteria – principally the fermenting bacteria *lactobacilli*. One of the criteria for its diagnosis is a positive 'whiff test', which involves placing a drop of potassium hydroxide on a swab of vaginal secretion. The unmistakable fishy smell of bacterial vaginosis is due to the presence of aromatic amines that include the colourfully named putrescine and cadaverine. BV is not considered to be a sexually transmitted infection, but it does appear to be more common among lesbians, suggesting that oral sex may have some role in its aetiology.

Some bacteria which normally live in the air can also adapt to the prevailing environmental conditions and live anaerobically. *Pseudomonas aeruginosa* is a hardy organism found just about anywhere, but it particularly likes to live in your sink, bath or shower. Human infection with this bug is rare in patients outside of hospital and usually only occurs in people who are immunosuppressed. When some strains of the bacterium cause an infection they produce green pus that has a fruity smell like a week-old dishcloth. The reason that a dishcloth smells that way is because it is saturated with, among other things, *Pseudomonas aeruginosa*. (Note to self: throw away week-old dishcloth tonight.)

But the worst medical smell I have encountered was associated with the severe disease of the genital and associated areas, donovanosis *(see chapter 11)*. In some places the condition was known as dead dog disease, and you only had to experience the smell to know why. However, the bug that causes donovanosis doesn't itself produce any discernible odour – it is what is known as super-infection with anaerobic bacteria that causes the stench. Sometimes after seeing a donovanosis patient in the morning I could smell it for the rest of the day.

Humans have evolved to find some smells unpleasant, so they avoid contact with the source, but awful as it may be, a smell itself is not immediately dangerous to an infectious diseases doctor. The same can't be said though for the microbiologist.

The amount of 'art' that is required in the microbiology laboratory would surprise the casual observer, who might be expecting a more cut-and-dried scientific approach to bacterial isolation. Lab scientists make hundreds of judgment calls every day. Is that little colony at the edge of the agar plate a contaminant or a pathogen? Is there a dangerous bug hiding underneath the overgrowth of what looks like harmless throat bacteria? Is that normal skin flora or a staphylococcus? There are millions of different bacteria, but only a few thousand are considered to be responsible for human disease. Deciding which is benign and which dangerous on an agar plate requires years of experience. When I was a student learning microbiology it was accepted practice that one of the ways to identify bacteria was to take a good deep whiff of the plate – a practice now officially forbidden for OH&S reasons because of the risk of transmitting a pathogen. (Indeed, at my medical school smelling a plate was allegedly responsible for a case of gonorrhoea of the throat in a female student. Her explanation was that she had picked up the infection during a laboratory session on sexually transmitted diseases. Her practical class partner, a young man known for his enthusiastic heterosexuality, remained gallantly silent throughout her ordeal.) Despite the official ban, however, older microbiologists can still be observed taking a furtive smell of a plate to confirm or refute their diagnostic suspicions.

Eternal sunshine of the spotless mind

The memory of a smell can be stored in several places in the brain – some of these anatomical sites are close to regions responsible for emotion and long-term memory. It is no surprise, then, that smell can trigger distant and otherwise indistinct memories. The best smell in the world, wet grass encrusting the underside of a lawn mower mixed with a hint of leaded petrol, is my father; this is my earliest memory of him and I must have been about three years old when it was first encoded into my brain's circuitry. A deep sense of contentment alternating with an almost over-whelming wistfulness overtakes me when I encounter it now. Another powerful activator for me is a sweet rubbery odour. I had smelt it intermittently for decades but was unable to pin-point the source until I eventually realised that it was the smell of the teat of a baby's bottle being sterilised in boiling water.

Recently in the hospital foyer I bumped into one of my HIV patients. I hadn't seen him in my clinic for 18 months and I was a little taken aback by his appearance. Even though he was an alcoholic, he was a professional man, usually well dressed and presentable, but since I had seen him last his cirrhosis had pro-gressed. He now had the thin arms, gaunt facial features, yellow eyes and swollen abdomen that is a 'full hand' for end-stage liver disease. I was sad to see his deterioration, but I wasn't ready for the smell that assaulted me when I stood next to him: I was surrounded by an effluvium of urine, foetor hepaticus and the ingrained remnants of tobacco smoke – the alcoholic's olfactory trifecta. The smell, so deeply embedded in my own cortex, took me spinning back in time to my days as a junior doctor. If my first surgical registrar had been with me he would have called this patient a 'dunny'.

A large proportion of my patients in my junior doctor days were homeless men and women, mainly alcoholics. A few of them were 'characters' who were quite good fun to interact with, but most were very sad or very mad, and essentially unreachable. They would turn up in the casualty department throughout the day and night, and I would sew up lacerations, bandage sprained limbs, plaster broken bones and, on occasion, get them ready for neurosurgery to remove a clot from around the brain. I became proficient in the management of end-stage liver disease and it wouldn't be until I was rotated to another hospital that I learnt that alcohol-related problems were actually a little exotic in the mainstream medical world.

The homeless were usually brought to the hospital after they had been found in trouble by the police or by the ambulance. They rarely wanted help, or offered thanks when it was provided. Their inability to look after themselves was often interpreted by the doctors and nurses as a conscious refusal to do so: the myth of the primacy of 'personal responsibility' ruled in some medical minds and legitimised their contempt for these patients.

Regardless of the sex, race or favourite drink of these patients, one thing was always the same: the rank combination of urine, tobacco and grime from cobblestones made them smell like a public urinal. So they were called dunnies. If you asked a colleague what the preceding night shift had been like, the response might be: 'Not too bad, just an infarct and a couple of dunnies'. I heard the term the moment I arrived as a student in 1980 and it seemed to be peculiar to our hospital; it was used by most of the resident staff but I never heard any of the consultants use it. In the beginning I thought that the word was harmless and I must have used it myself a few times. One day, however, I witnessed a registrar being spoken to by one of the nuns.

'I never want to hear you speak of any of our patients in that way', she said in a quiet voice. There was never any dissent when a nun spoke and a reprimand of this nature was uncommon and devastating. Such a public censure pushed the word further underground, but it did not disappear.

What drives those who have chosen a career that is supposed to be about caring to demean some of the recipients of that care? Every medical culture does it. *The House of God*, a 1970s novel about a Boston intern, popularised the term 'gomer' – short for 'Get Out of My Emergency Room' – which described a similar group of hapless and/or obnoxious patients. But dunny was worse: we were not just saying you smell *like* a toilet (because that was true) but that you *are* a toilet. The paradox was that our hospital really did reach out to the homeless and prided itself on its equity of access. Other hospitals would probably have been far less tolerant in admitting down-and-outs and the homeless.

Young doctors always buffer the real stresses of their work with humour that may not seem appropriate to the uninitiated, but I think with dunny they went too far, and even at this distance I am embarrassed by the memory. What we call people, regardless of our underlying motivation, can determine the way we treat them. Today most of the intolerance that I observe in medical staff is directed at patients who inject drugs: most hold quietly intolerant opinions (although the publicly proffered attitude of some senior colleagues would make you question their right to hold the title 'doctor').The injecting drug user is sometimes a 'junkie' or 'addict', but it is the behaviour of the staff that betrays their feelings. Some doctors refuse to take these patients' symptoms seriously, occasionally with the disastrous consequences of delayed and missed diagnoses.

I made a decision never to call anyone a dunny after I overheard the registrar's dressing-down and I made sure that no one who worked under my supervision subsequently did either. We should not be afraid of trying to change the culture of our workplaces. Sometimes we just need someone to tell us that we can.

11

Like a blowtorch to the groin

Klebsiella granulomatis – a Gram-negative bacterium that causes the sexually transmitted infection, donovanosis. Previously known as *Calymmatobacter granulomatis*, the organism is unable to be grown in the laboratory using routine culture techniques. *K. granulomatis* has not attracted the attention of the international research community in the way that other more marketable sexually transmitted infections, such as genital herpes, have. Once common in the Northern Territory and remote parts of Western Australia and Queensland, donovanosis has now nearly disappeared from Australia.

'People are usually more convinced by reasons they discovered themselves than by those found by others.' (Blaise Pascal, 1623–1662)

A few weeks before moving to the Northern Territory in 1992, I sat in the Fairfield Infectious Diseases Hospital library reading a copy of Stephen Morse's *Atlas of Sexually Transmitted Diseases and AIDS*. I had recently completed my training as an infectious diseases physician and because my special area of interest had been HIV I thought of myself principally as an AIDS doctor. I'd had little opportunity to get much specific experience in sexually transmitted infections and I was fast coming to the realisation that I would need to learn a lot more about them if I was to be of any use in my new position as co-ordinator of the Northern Territory's AIDS and STD programs for the health department in Darwin.

The medical atlas is to medicine what the graphic novel is to post-modern literature: an easy way to tap into a body of knowledge without having to commit to all the hard bits – such as text. Richard Feynman – the great 20th century physicist and bongo drums player, who probably knew more about how the sub-atomic world worked than any other person living at the time – was almost dismissive of the naming of things. He said that he could know the name of a bird in every language in the world and still know nothing whatever about the bird. He wanted to look at the bird and see what it was doing. He didn't mean that taxonomy isn't important – without it there is no chance of developing grander theories – just that there was a difference between knowing the name of something and knowing something. Feynman's comments resonated with me (albeit the harmonics occurring in a brain several orders of magnitude less powerful than Feynman's). I like to know what the boundaries of knowledge in a particular field are; where the limits to understanding are. I like to bring the camera into wide-angle rather than tight close-up.

I was leafing through Morse's work when I reached a chapter titled 'Granuloma inguinale'. Now here was something that I not only knew nothing about but had never even heard of. There was another condition with a similar name that I was aware of – lymphogranuloma venereum or LGV – but this was caused by *Chlamydia trachomatis*, a bug that I knew quite a lot about *(see chapter 13)*.

It turned out that, like many rare diseases, granuloma inguinale suffered from nominal instability – its name had changed many times since its first description by a British surgeon in India in 1882. The disease had been referred to as 'ulcerating granuloma of the pudenda', 'granuloma venereum', 'granuloma tropicum', 'chronic venereal sore' and, eponymously, as 'dono-vanosis', after Major Charles Donovan, who first identified the causative organism in 1905 in Madras (since subject to a name change of its own – the city is now known as Chennai). The disease was confined to a limited number of geographical regions: southern Africa, parts of India and the Caribbean, New Guinea and northern Australia.

You develop a strong stomach for horrible images as a doctor but as I looked at the pictures and read the descriptions that accompanied them in Morse's book, I found myself crossing my legs in sympathy for the sufferers. I learnt that the disease principally affects the genital region of both men and women, producing lumps and nodules that can progress to ulcers and eventually to genital destruction. The pictures were like nothing I had seen before. The infection could start on the skin of the genitals or infect the cervix and spread up through the uterus to involve the tissues surrounding the ovaries and kidneys. It could infect the ear canal of children born to an infected mother, and there were case reports of the disease occurring in most parts of the body. Because the name 'inguinale' means situated in the groin, hence failing to capture the disease's anatomic reach, many authorities preferred to call it donovanosis.

The disease is caused by a bacterium that, in the early 1990s, was called *Calymmatobacterium granulomatis* – a germ known to very few microbiologists. It belonged to a genus of its own – there were no other calymmatobacters. The organism liked to live within human cells, was not easily grown in the laboratory, and its genetic structure was completely unknown. The *Atlas* said that it had last been cultured in 1962 and there was no laboratory that had the expertise to work on it.

The disease was considered to be sexually transmitted, although many who contracted it had no history of having an infected sexual partner. It was, however, known to have been transmitted following rape, and it did not occur in people who had never been sexually active, except in the case of babies born to mothers with an infected birth canal. Donovanosis could be treated with antibiotics, but they had to be administered for several weeks to ensure a cure.

I closed the book, almost immediately forgot the name of the bug and knew that I would probably confuse granuloma inguinale and lymphogranuloma venereum with each other if anyone, for some strange reason, should ever ask.

From pictures to the real thing

About six months later I was asked to see an Aboriginal man in the Royal Darwin Hospital. He had been brought up from the hospital in Katherine because of an ulcer in his groin. As I walked onto the ward and introduced myself to the patient, I remember thinking that it was a little extravagant to transport someone over 300 kilometres because of an ulcer. He was in his 40s, admitted to drinking 'a lot of alcohol' and at some time in the unspecified past he had noticed a lump 'down there' which had got worse with time. I asked if I could have a look, and without hesitation he pulled back the sheets. I hope that my face did not betray my shock at what I saw: he was wearing nothing and I could see that his entire groin region was an open, weeping sore that smelt like rotting meat. It looked like someone had applied a blow torch to his genitals. The tip of his penis still had skin, but on the shaft and scrotum the skin seemed to have been burnt away. The ulceration extended through his perineum to involve a strip of skin around his anus.

Despite the extent of the tissue involved, he didn't seem to be in too much discomfort and he was not unwell: he had no fever, there was no evidence of any inflammation of the skin beyond the edges of the groin lesions, and he was actually reasonably bright and cheery. I looked at his medical chart – mainly because

I needed an excuse to look somewhere else for a moment – and I noted that the swabs from his groin had grown a mixture of organisms that would be unlikely to cause this kind of illness. The doctors in Katherine had put him on intravenous antibiotics and made a provisional diagnosis of donovanosis. There was no history of contact with anyone else with the disease. Getting an accurate sexual history is difficult even with the most liberated and worldly patient; with an Aboriginal man constrained by complex cultural proprieties the chances of obtaining accurate information about sexual partners at the initial consultation were minimal. From the notes it appeared that his current state was actually an improvement on when he was first seen a week previously. He had been sent to Darwin for consideration of skin grafting. I asked my registrar to perform a biopsy of the ulcer and I wrote in the notes that I agreed with the diagnosis and that antibiotics should continue for a further four weeks. I realised that it was time for me to really learn about this disease.

In the first few weeks of my new job I had been told by a number of colleagues that if I needed to know anything about some of the more exotic STIs in the Territory then there was only one thing to do: 'Speak to H. He knows more about donovanosis and gonorrhoea and syphilis than anyone in the Top End'. H. was a communicable diseases nurse who worked in East Arnhem Land, based in the mining town of Nhulunbuy (or Gove as it was originally called). After seeing the patient from Katherine I gave him a call. His speech had the slow tempo and broad vowels of the north Queenslander and it was soon apparent that he had the patience to instruct the wet-behind-the-ears southerner at the other end of the telephone. H. was a local legend. In addition to his full-time job with the Territory health department, he was a voluntary pilot for a missionary organisation that had provided services to the Top End for a generation, and he was well known in all the Aboriginal communities in the area. He was an expert in tuberculosis and leprosy and had seen things that few, if any other, medical persons in Australia ever will. He fished in, and swam in, crocodile-infested rivers, with his children in tow, but always got out when he 'felt the electricity in the water' that told him a crocodile was nearby. He had driven his old four-wheel-drive to places that no white person had ever been, and had more near-misses in his light plane than an air force test pilot. He had, as they say, no tickets on himself, and he maintained an air of humility and graciousness in the face of the undeniable chaos of the local health scene.

'If you look up the books they say that donovanosis only occurs in the Top End', he told me. 'We see a dozen or so cases over here each year, but there's more cases in central Australia than up here. They just don't publish anything in the journals down there, so it never gets into the textbooks.' He quoted a recent review article in an international journal on STIs which had included a global map of the distribution of the disease. This indicated that there was no donovanosis south of Katherine. 'It's very difficult to cure because people stop taking the antibiotics after a few days. But if you get the antibiotics in, they'll get better.'

A few years before I arrived in Darwin one of the doctors there, Angela Merianos, had conducted a trial which showed that daily antibiotic injections could cure donovanosis. But this regimen was not an easy thing to organise – sometimes it was necessary to admit the patient to hospital to ensure that the treatment was administered. There was no intrinsic benefit of an injection over oral antibiotics, it was just a way of ensuring that the patient received the drug.

'They say it's sexually transmitted but I'm not so sure', continued H. 'I've seen it in old men who haven't had a wife for years and in old women whose husbands have died. I reckon it's got something to do with genital hygiene.' I thanked him for his advice, of which I would receive much more over the next eight years.

The biopsy from the Aboriginal patient confirmed the diagnosis of donovanosis. Using the special stain necessary, the bacteria, known as Donovan bodies, could be seen as tiny safety pin-like rods inside the collections of white blood cells that had migrated to the ulcer to try to control the infection. Even an experienced pathologist may need to spend half an hour looking through a biopsy to find one cluster of Donovan bodies, but this tissue sample was teeming with them. Cancers can develop in any chronic ulcer and the association of malignancy and donovanosis was well described in the old literature that I was now starting to read with growing interest. There was no evidence of cancer in this biopsy so we had the confidence to continue the treatment and to hold off on skin-grafting. After a few more days of giving the man an intravenous antibiotic we changed the treatment to an oral one and kept him in hospital until his skin had completely healed. By the time he was ready to leave, his groin was scarred and de-pigmented and he had lost the ability to have an erection. When he was first admitted, however, he'd thought that he was dying, so he didn't appear to be fazed too much by the limitations of the result – indeed, he was effusive in his thanks to the medical and nursing teams. He had been in hospital for nearly three months.

From curiosity towards clarification

The Menzies School of Health Research in Darwin is one of Australia's leading research institutions for Aboriginal and tropical health. In 1993 it was still in its first decade and lacked a permanent home. Offices were located on the first floor of the old nurses' home at Royal Darwin Hospital, and the school's scientists vied for space in the hospital's microbiological laboratory. Menzies, as it was always known locally, was a broad church, and nurtured activities across the social, biological and clinical sciences. There were programs relating to epidemiology, anthropology, molecular biology, infectious diseases, substance abuse, renal disease and ear health, to name a few. Seminars were held by the school every Friday afternoon, and these attracted the city's small audience of researchers, along with other interested people. I was employed by the health department but I worked closely with a number of Menzies people. One Friday afternoon, a senior member of the school, a microbiologist, presented a paper on 'interesting infections' and included donovanosis as a small part of the talk – a 'curiosity'. By then I had seen a few more cases myself and I was starting to appreciate how much more common the terrible consequences of the disease might be than was implied by the paper's presenter.

It is axiomatic that STIs cause few or no symptoms in the majority of the people that they infect. For example, fewer than 10 per cent of those who are infected with herpes simplex type 2 virus *(see chapter 10)* ever develop clinically apparent genital herpes. Genital chlamydia *(see chapter 13)* remains a public health issue because the vast majority of the thousands of young women who contract it every year are unaware that they are infected (the disease slowly, and painlessly, causes scarring of their fallopian tubes, so that when they find themselves infertile later in life they may never realise that it was an undiagnosed chlamydial infection years before that was responsible). In contrast, donovanosis causes most of its damage immediately: some of the handful of patients that I had seen up to that point had rapidly developed the horrible, disfiguring lesions on their penis or vulva, forcing them to withdraw from society.

I sat at that Friday afternoon talk with a medical colleague, Ivan Bastian, who was just finishing his doctoral thesis at Menzies. Afterwards, we started talking about the issues that we should address in regard to this awful, if fascinating, disease. We agreed that the epidemiology of the disease needed to be clarified. Epidemiology (literally, 'the study of what is upon people') is the cornerstone of all medicine. It sets about answering a number of crucial questions. Who has the disease – men or women, the young or the old? What are the factors that determine infection? Is the disease limited to a specific geographical location or population? What happens to people who are infected (what is the natural history of the disease)? We take the epidemiology of most diseases for granted. For instance, it seems self-evident that lung cancer is caused by smoking, but it wasn't always so. Before British epidemiologist Sir Richard Doll's famous study in the 1950s demonstrated that smokers were about 13 times more likely to contract lung cancer than non-smokers, no link had been made between the habit and the disease. Even then the information did not really enter into public health consciousness until the 1960s, and was criminally denied by the tobacco industry for another two decades. Only such epidemiological studies can give the clues to how to control disease, and such research requires time and effort. The only Australian information at the beginning of the 1990s about who was getting donovanosis and where they lived came from the National Notifiable Diseases System database, held in Canberra.

Many, but not all, infectious diseases are 'notifiable'. Measles, mumps and rubella virus infections are, golden staph, streptococcal and *E. coli* infections are not. A disease usually becomes notifiable if there is a vaccine available for it or if there is a recognised public health intervention, such as tracing contacts in the case of people with STIs or closing restaurants in the case of outbreaks of food poisoning. Once a disease is on the list every new diagnosis must be relayed to a central collection point. The states and territories individually collect certain information and channel it to Canberra, where it is collated and analysed. There are many inherent weaknesses in this data – although it is mandated by law to provide the information, in reality its completeness relies upon the goodwill of the participating laboratories and individual practitioners who diagnose the diseases in question. Laboratory notifications are always more reliable than practitioner notifications: strange as it may sound, filling in a form and sending it to a health department is not the highest thing on most doctors' priority list.

Confirmation of a diagnosis of donovanosis required a positive finding of the characteristic Donovan bodies in a biopsy specimen. We knew that doctors and nurses working in remote areas were reluctant to perform biopsies (or hadn't been trained to do so) and that patients didn't like the sound of the procedure when it was offered. As a result, most cases of donovanosis were diagnosed on the basis of the clinical appearances alone. The national database showed that in 1993 there were 36 cases of donovanosis notified in the Northern Territory, 14 in Queensland and 38 in Western Australia. All of the cases occurred in Aboriginal people, and they ranged from the young to the elderly. Two of my registrars sent out questionnaires to all practitioners who could conceivably diagnose donovanosis in the Northern Territory, asking them if they had seen any cases in the previous 12 months. As a result, 119 cases of donovanosis that had been treated in the Northern Territory in 1993 were identified, demonstrating that the official data underestimated the true number of patients by a factor of about three. Extrapolating this to Queensland and Western Australia, we estimated that there were about 300 cases of donovanosis across Australia each year.

So here was an important lesson: a disease that I had never heard of two years previously, which had no profile in mainstream textbooks and which was certainly not on any local public health priority list, was infecting about 300 Aboriginal people each year and causing serious illness, and a loss of self-esteem or, as Territory Aboriginals called it, 'shame'. The disease was treatable with antibiotics and should have been easy to detect because it always produced visible symptoms. So why was it still present in Aboriginal Australia but not in White Australia? And why did nobody seem particularly interested outside of the small number of local clinicians who struggled to treat it? We published the results of the study in *Venereology*, an Australian journal that did not appear on Medline, the National Library of Medicine's electronic database. It was therefore 'invisible' to the international medical community. Attempts to get local widespread coverage misfired when I gave a long interview to the *NT News*, describing donovanosis in some detail to a cub reporter – and, as it turned out, creating the wrong impression. When I went down to the newsagent's to pick up the newspaper, a picture of me in my office was plastered across the front page under the headline 'Strange Sex Bug Hits the NT'. It takes a lot to bump a crocodile story from the front page of the *NT News*, so I should take some solace.

It is possible that donovanosis was introduced into the Top End by Macassan traders who had been in contact with coastal Aboriginal populations since the 16th century – hundreds of years before British colonisation. In 1898 the chief health officer of the Northern Territory, a Dr Goldsmith, received from Britain a copy of the first edition of Manson's *Tropical Diseases*. Reading it, Goldsmith noticed that certain types of genital lesions seen in Africa were similar to those he had observed in local Aboriginal patients. He wrote to Manson, commenting that mercury and potassium iodide (then used to treat syphilis) were ineffectual. At the Intercolonial Medical Congress of Australasia in 1899 Goldsmith presented a paper on 'Ulcerating Granuloma of the Pudenda' in which he stated that the disease occurred in both sexes and 'in Europeans, Asiatics and aboriginals'. He believed it to be venereal in nature and to be only mildly contagious. When Donovan identified the organisms that caused the disease in 1905 it became possible to differentiate it from syphilis, but a letter to the *Australasian Medical Gazette* in 1911 showed that the disease was still commonly confused with syphilis in northern Australia.

An extraordinary epidemic of donovanosis occurred in the Marind-Anim people of New Guinea in the first part of the

20th century. It has been estimated that 10 000 people out of a total population of 15 000 were affected over a 20-year period. Consistent with the international and time-honoured practice of blaming someone else for an epidemic of sexually transmitted infection, it was claimed that the disease had been introduced by Aboriginal labourers who had been brought from Australia to build a station in the early 1900s.

In 1910 the arsenic-based compound arsphenamine (trade name, Salvarsan) was used to treat syphilis – the first time an infectious disease had been effectively cured with an antimicrobial compound *(see page 24)*. The second condition would be donovanosis, when, in 1913, Brazilian researchers demonstrated the value of intravenous potassium antimonyl tartrate in the treatment of the disease. Despite its considerable toxicity, the heavy metal compound was used extensively in New Guinea and is credited with controlling the Marind-Anim epidemic. The agent was first used in Australia in 1922 to treat 30 cases of donovanosis in Darwin.

After the Second World War officers in the Northern Territory medical services described donovanosis as a fairly common disease of the Aboriginal male, accounting for 3.3 per cent of hospital admissions to the Aboriginal ward in Darwin Hospital. When antibiotics became available their improved efficacy and safety quickly consigned potassium antimonyl tartrate (and arsphenamine) to history. In 1953 the first reports of the successful treatment of donovanosis with the anti-TB drug streptomycin were published.

Donovanosis was well described in poor blacks in the southern states of the USA in the early 20th century, but by the 1960s the disease had completely disappeared. (Donovanosis-containing material was used in transmission experiments as part of the infamous Tuskegee syphilis experiments in the USA, when its low infectivity and the difficulty of growing it using routine laboratory techniques were demonstrated.) By 1990, Australia was the last developed country in the world where the disease was still endemic – albeit restricted to one section of the population.

The decline of a disease in the developed world means that research interest in it wanes and there is little or no subsequent progress in its management or diagnosis. It happened to tuberculosis in the two decades after the Second World War: as the disease disappeared from the industrialised nations due to screening with chest X-rays and treatment with antibiotics, interest in vaccine and pharmaceutical research faded to a point where there was virtually no advance in the treatment of the disease for a generation. The only currently available vaccine for TB is BCG (Bacillus Calmette-Guérin) – one that would never be licensed today because of its low efficacy. It has only been in the last decade, because of the emergence of multiple-drug-resistant TB, and thanks to funding from the Bill and Melinda Gates Foundation, that interest in discovering a vaccine for TB has resurged. The cynic could argue that the main reason is not concern for the welfare of people in the developing world, where the disease is endemic, but the threat that incurable TB poses to the West. If you subscribe to that explanation, it is not surprising that donovanosis, which only affected small, marginalised and scattered populations, should have been so neglected by the medical mainstream.

When we undertook the study seeking information on the real number of cases of donovanosis in the Northern Territory, we asked the doctors and nurses what they believed to be the most important barriers to its control. The most commonly cited reason for failure of treatment was the need to continue the antibiotics for at least a month. Most patients, it was reported, would take the treatment for a while – usually long enough for the antibiotics to bring the ulceration and the smell under control – and then they would stop, allowing the disease to recur. It was clear that a better regimen of treatment was needed.

A new drug

Around that time, John Mathews, the director of Menzies, was interested in a new antibiotic for the treatment of the eye disease trachoma. It had been licensed but was not yet released on the Australian market. The drug, azithromycin, was chemically related to a frequently prescribed antibiotic, erythromycin, but azithromycin had the advantage of only needing to be given once a day instead of four times, and it was associated with fewer side-effects. Furthermore, because it was taken up by the white blood cells that migrate to sites of infection and released where it was most needed, azithromycin's ability to become concentrated in human body tissues was far greater than that of other antibiotics. While it sounded to me like an ideal candidate for the treatment of donovanosis, there was a much more pressing and less speculative role for the drug.

Azithromycin was being used overseas for the treatment of genital chlamydial infections – a single dose was as good as a week to ten days' of treatment with tetracycline antibiotics – but there was little interest from the Australian venereological community and the pharmaceutical company that sponsored azithromycin had no immediate plans to market the drug here. The barriers to the treatment of chlamydia in Aboriginal populations were similar to those in the case of donovanosis, and so I obtained funding through the Commonwealth Department of Health to import 1000 doses of azithromycin from the USA for use in the Northern Territory. We were the first group in Australia to use the drug to treat chlamydia. The antibiotic was very effective, well tolerated by patients and dramatically simplified chlamydia treatment. And my friends took considerable pleasure in congratulating me in my new role as drug importer.

Ivan and I agreed that we should design a trial to investigate the use of azithromycin for the treatment of donovanosis. We would investigate the effectiveness of two different regimens: a single dose once a week for four weeks and a single dose once a day for seven days. We decided that we would only include patients who had an unequivocal diagnosis – patients had to have a positive biopsy before they could be included in the trial. We needed permission from two regional ethics committees before we could start.

Some researchers find the process of obtaining ethics clearance unnecessarily time-consuming and even obstructive. While there is no doubt that the processes could be streamlined and that committees can occasionally make decisions that seem unreasonable, the writing of an ethics submission gives the researcher a chance to fine-tune the study's methodology and to anticipate some (but never all) of the possible problems that could arise in the course of the research. One of the main ethical issues to be considered was that we could not run laboratory tests first because we could not culture the disease and no animal models existed for testing. In addition, the committee was aware that currently available antibiotics *would* work if the patients could be supervised adequately for a long period of time. The clinicians on the committee who had experience with donovanosis were aware that the latter was extremely difficult, and with some minor amendments the protocol was approved. We waited for our first patient.

It wasn't long before one of the district medical officers notified us of a 20-year-old man with a large, red, raised penile lesion that was visible when he retracted his foreskin. He had been identified as a result of contact-tracing after his girlfriend was diagnosed with donovanosis of the cervix. Because of our limited experience with azithromycin, we had to be extremely strict about who could receive it. Early reports had suggested that the inner ear could be damaged by high doses of the drug, and when we found that our first potential recruit wore a hearing aid we had to exclude him from the study (these fears have not been realised in patients who receive the standard doses of azithromycin and today he would receive treatment). Instead, we supervised the prolonged, but ultimately successful, treatment of the man and his girlfriend with the standard antibiotics – it took a month.

Our next patient was an old lady from a remote community who had come to the attention of the nursing staff at the local health clinic because she had trouble walking – a most unusual presentation of donovanosis, it would have to be admitted. By the time we saw her she was using crutches and had what are known as kissing ulcers – two identical lesions on each labium majora (the lips of the vagina). These ulcers would partly heal and join together in the process of forming scar tissue, effectively sealing the entry to her vagina, but if she walked the scab would tear, causing pain and bleeding. A biopsy confirmed the diagnosis of donovanosis, the trial was described to her, and after a good hour of discussion she gave us written consent to be enrolled in the study. She was randomised to receive a 500mg dose of azithromycin once a day for seven days. The plan was to watch her closely for signs of healing and to change her to the usual antibiotics if she did not respond to the new drug. We gave the patient her first dose and the nurse in her home clinic was organised to give the subsequent doses. She would be seen by us again in seven days. It was a long week.

I almost didn't recognise her when she returned to the clinic. The crutches were gone and she strode down the clinic corridor, taking long, obviously painless steps. She smiled at me, and I thought for a moment that she was going to hug me. When I examined her I saw that the lesions were showing definite signs of healing: it was clear that azithromycin worked at least to some degree at this dose. A week later the woman was back and the lesions had nearly completely healed. We were starting to get more confident about the antibiotic's effectiveness but we needed more patients before we could be sure.

Over the next months we enrolled a further ten patients with confirmed donovanosis for the study and every one of them responded rapidly and completely. The most exciting finding was that a dose of one gram (two capsules) once a week for four weeks appeared to be as effective as seven consecutive days at the same dose. The advantage of the weekly dosing was that it could be used for patients in the bush – the time interval made it practical for a supervised dose to be administered by overstretched health services in remote areas. Eleven patients successfully treated was only a start – but we now knew that we had an effective and safe new antibiotic treatment that could be used in a campaign to control donovanosis. Steve Skov, a doctor then working in Alice Springs, ran a study to explore the use of azithromycin under real-world conditions. His trial ultimately enrolled more than 50 patients, including one old man who had been prescribed other antibiotics on 90 occasions but had never been cured. The results could not have been more compelling: there were no treatment failures and Steve showed, for the first time, that effective treatment of donovanosis in the field was feasible. As a result of these two studies, the WHO and the US Centers for Disease Control added azithromycin to their guidelines for the treatment of donovanosis, although the WHO guidelines recommend one gram on the first day of treatment and then 500 milligrams daily until the lesions have healed. Our studies showed that just seven days of treatment led to a cure in all cases – regardless of the extent of the lesions. It is unclear how the WHO arrived at its recommendation.

A new test and a new name

Calymmatobacterium granulomatis, the name given to the bacterium that caused donovanosis, had last been cultured in the laboratory in 1962 in the USA, which was also around the time that the disease disappeared in that country. The published method of culture involved inoculation of bacteria into the yolk sacs of chickens' eggs. This was a common method for culturing many species of bacteria in the 1960s, but with the advent of modern cell culture techniques it had become a rarely performed procedure. Because *C. granulomatis* could not be cultured in the lab by the contemporary methods, Ivan Bastian taught himself the technique used in America 30 years earlier. He procured the requisite eggs and attempted to culture the organism from a number of specimens collected from donovanosis patients. Although there were some promising results, the method was time-consuming and cumbersome, and after a number of attempts Ivan gave up. Early on during these experiments, Sue Hutton, another Menzies scientist, suggested in the tea room one morning that we should use the method that she employed to culture chlamydia. For some reason we didn't take her advice.

In the early 1990s a diagnostic procedure called PCR – which stands for polymerase chain reaction – was fast becoming the scientific plat du jour. Invented by the eccentric Kari Mullis, who won the Nobel Prize for its discovery, PCR allowed tiny amounts of DNA to be amplified in the laboratory. The power of this technique is astounding and was originally explained to me this way …

Imagine taking a drop of a sample containing the DNA that you want to measure and putting it in an Olympic-size swimming pool. Then after the water in the pool has been mixed up by, say, a swimming competition, you take a drop out of the pool and place it in another Olympic pool. Stir. Take a drop out of this second pool and, using PCR, you will be able to identify the sequence of the DNA that you put into the first swimming pool.

A major advantage of PCR was that it could be performed on a simple surface swab of a suspicious lesion, thus avoiding the need for a biopsy, which we knew was a problem for both patients and clinicians. Furthermore, DNA is surprisingly stable during transport and it would mean that a specimen could be transported from a remote area under hot, dry or humid conditions and a reliable result could still be expected. The benefits that PCR testing would bring to our battle against donovanosis were obvious.

As well as the practical advance of being able to make a diagnosis of donovanosis in the lab, the advent of PCR also allowed Ivan to pursue a related matter. He had become convinced that *C. granulomatis* was not the sole species of an exclusive genus, but really belonged to the family *Klebsiellae*, bacteria well known to microbiologists as causes of urinary tract infections and pneumonia. To test his hunch he designed a set of PCR primers (small molecules that latch onto the bacterium's DNA sequence) to target a gene that was likely to be present in the bacterium if it truly was a klebsiella. The experiment worked and, after confirming the result on a number of specimens, Ivan had enough evidence to support his hypothesis.

In 1995 Ivan's work took him away from the Northern Territory, but Dave Kemp, the deputy director of Menzies and one of Australia's legends of molecular biology, maintained an interest in the development of PCR. Over the next few years, another scientist, Jenny Carter, worked with Dave and Sri Sriprakash to develop a simple PCR system for the diagnosis of donovanosis. Soon we had a functioning in-house PCR kit that could be used by doctors and nurses in the bush when they collected a swab. Jenny was also the first person to culture the bug in Australia, having been just beaten to the mark by a South African group who were also interested in donovanosis. The technique she used was the one that Sue Hutton had suggested several years earlier (Sue very generously refrained from ever saying I told you so). Although this was an extremely exciting event for all of us, the cell culture method was still time-consuming and fiddly and was quickly overtaken by the PCR.

The continuing experiments with PCR expanded information about the molecular make-up of the donovanosis bacterium, and soon Jenny Carter proved that Ivan's hunch was correct: the bug was definitely a member of the family *Klebsiellae*. Jenny published the findings in the *International Journal of Systematic Bacteriology*, the arbiter of bacterial classification. The journal accepted the paper for publication and as a result *Calymmatobacterium granulomatis* was officially renamed *Klebsiella granulomatis*. We all felt like proud godparents. I still do.

Towards an eradication campaign

By now we knew where donovanosis occurred in Australia, we had a diagnostic method that could identify it easily and accurately, and we could prescribe an effective and safe antibiotic for its treatment. These were the ingredients for a control program.

Through a Commonwealth-funded collaboration between public health units in South Australia, the Northern Territory and Western Australia called the Tri-State Project, dozens of people in central Australia with donovanosis were identified and cured employing the simple, traditional public health approach of increasing awareness, facilitating diagnosis and assisting with treatment. In 1996, with the success of the central Australian project in mind, I approached the then federal minister for health, Michael Wooldridge, with the idea of a national donovanosis eradication campaign. I sought support from all the key players in the regions where the disease was endemic and secured it, with one important exception – one of the Aboriginal-controlled health services in the Northern Territory – which was a pity because the Aboriginal-controlled services in other areas of northern Australia had given their imprimatur. As a result, the initial momentum was lost and it would take another five years of Wooldridge's quiet patronage for the idea to turn into funding. In 2000 the Office of Aboriginal and Torres Strait Islander Health (OATSIH), part of the Department of

Health and Ageing, was asked to fund a program and form a committee to oversee an eradication campaign. Bernie Pearce from OATSIH was the driving force behind the program and he asked me to chair the Donovanosis Eradication Committee, which was composed of representatives of the State and Territory governments and regional Aboriginal Health Services, and experts in clinical, laboratory and epidemiological matters. The plan was simple: four nurses would be employed, based in Perth, Cairns, Darwin and Alice Springs; they would report to their local health departments over day-to-day issues but to the committee over strategic and technical matters.

The official launch of the campaign took place at the annual National HIV Conference in 2000 and ran for two years. By its conclusion the number of cases of donovanosis had fallen to its lowest level since data was first collected. From a peak of 121 officially notified cases in Australia in 1994, only one case was reported in 2009. No other STI in Australia has shown such a decline and fall in the past 50 years.

A degree of disillusionment

I had a large portion of my naivety removed without anaesthetic by the politicking and red tape involved in getting the eradication campaign off the ground, so I wasn't surprised by what happened next. As the success of the program became increasingly clear I proposed to OATSIH that the model could be applied to a more common, and arguably more important, STI affecting Aboriginal people – syphilis. But it didn't happen and I subsequently learnt that from the outset non-Aboriginal advisers in the community sector had privately questioned the value of the donovanosis campaign, yet had been unsuccessful in their attempts to 'white-ant' it. However, once there was no direct high-level ministerial patronage to buffer their objections, these critics were able to convince OATSIH to treat the campaign as a one-off rather than as a template for new activity.

Here, then, is what the Second National Sexually Transmissible Infections Strategy 2010–2013 has to say in relation to Aboriginal and Torres Strait Islander people:

> … chlamydia rates generally increased between 2004 and 2008, with the exception of South Australia where they decreased. There was also an increase in rates of gonorrhoea in 2008, which are 36 times that for the non-Indigenous population. Infectious syphilis increased in the period 2004–08, although jurisdiction trends vary and in 2008 remain up to 15 times higher … than the rest of the Australian population … The continuing decline in the number of diagnoses of donovanosis, from 10 in 2004 to two in 2008, *may be a consequence of a coordinated response around improved diagnosis and treatment* (my italics)…

A linked national strategy, the Third National Aboriginal and Torres Strait Islander Blood Borne Virus and Sexually Transmissible Infections Strategy 2010–2013, does not even contain the word donovanosis. Both strategies contain the following recommendations about syphilis:

> … a jurisdiction-led response that strengthens comprehensive sexual health programs in the primary care setting … This response may include strategies to be detailed in implementation plans to improve syphilis testing, contact tracing and follow up, as well as health-provider and community education.

These are noble and appropriate goals but are no different from what has been proposed for 20 years.

Sometimes in public health you just have to be brave. This was obviously not one of those times. After its completion, a thorough, independent evaluation of the donovanosis eradication campaign was prepared. I realise it is cliché to say this, but since it is literally true, I will: the report sat on a shelf.

12

So common it can't be
a disease

Trichomonas vaginalis – a sexually transmitted protozoan parasite found in the vagina in women and the urethra in men. The organism possesses tail-like appendages called flagella which beat rhythmically to propel it through bodily fluids. In the mid-1900s it affected up to 40 per cent of people in industrialised countries. Today, over 200 million cases of trichomoniasis occur every year, mainly in the developing world. The disease is virtually eradicated from developed countries, though it lingers in disadvantaged populations.

'I go three, maybe four times a year to get tested … Most of the time I don't even need to. I just go for peace of mind.' (Kelly Osbourne, 1984–)

As far as microscopic organisms go, *Trichomonas vaginalis* is actually pretty big. In 1838, a French scientist called Alfred Donné reported seeing a strange organism swimming in fluid that he had collected from a woman with 'inflammation of the vagina'. The bug dwarfed the fuzzy little bacteria that were just visible to his then state-of-the-art microscope. Looking like a Lilliputian stingray, the organism, propelled by the tail-like flagella at its base, moved around the drop of fluid on his glass slide. Donné did not make a connection between the symptoms that the woman had presented with and the obviously living organism that he saw under his microscope. Over half-a-century later, in 1894, the organism would be found in secretions from a man's urethra, but it wouldn't be until 1915 that the parasite would be considered as a possible cause of urethritis (inflammation of the urethra).

For the next 40 years there would be debate about whether it was a cause of disease at all – until the 1950s, when in the USA a number of 'volunteers' with syphilis-related dementia had their urethras inoculated with the organism to see whether it caused symptoms. When the symptoms did arise in a proportion of these men, the next question was whether the infection was sexually transmitted. So many people in the United States and the United Kingdom had been diagnosed with trichomoniasis in the 1940s, many believed that it must be transmissible by means other than sex. An English microbiologist, one Dr J Whittington, was especially interested in how the infection spread and devised an ingenious experiment to test her hypothesis that the organism could be caught from a public toilet. She rigged up the seat in the women's toilet of her London clinic so that if one of her patients who had just been diagnosed with trichomoniasis went to pass urine an alarm would be triggered. Dr Whittington would rush into the cubicle – after the patient had left, it is hoped – swab the seat and see if she could find the parasite in the tiny amounts of urine gathered. And indeed she could! There were pathogens under her microscope in four out of the 11 samples that she collected. This finding prompted another British doctor to write a letter to the British medical journal, The Lancet, in 1953, in which he contended that the majority of cases of trichomoniasis were caught from public toilets. He argued for the mandatory adoption of the 'gap' toilet seat (one that doesn't join at the front and looks like a giant horseshoe) and warned that unless they were installed in all British public toilets as a matter of public health urgency the control of trichomoniasis in the realm would be impossible. (One reason that this clarion call was not immediately taken up by the medical world may have been that the letter was published in the same month that Watson and Crick reported their discovery of the structure of DNA.)

Tumble to extinction sets a riddle

It is hard to believe how common trichomoniasis was in the general population in the middle of the 20th century. In 1948 one expert estimated that up to one in five women in the USA were infected and a 1970 survey there showed that 10 per cent of white women and 30 per cent of black women who underwent a Pap smear (named after its inventor, the Greek doctor Georgios Papanikolaou) had trichomoniasis – though some disputed this finding. This prevalence declined a little over the next 30 years in the USA: a 1998 study showed 7 per cent of white or Hispanic women and 23 per cent of black women attending an antenatal clinic were infected. But over the same period in the United Kingdom, Australia and most European countries, the disease did something quite unexpected – it almost completely disappeared. In 1979, 18 per cent of women who attended an Australian STI clinic had trichomoniasis, but by the year 2000 the condition was simply not seen in urban STI clinics. And a UK study in 1998 showed only 0.1 per cent of Pap smears had evidence of the pathogen. What was going on?

T. vaginalis (frequently abbreviated to 'trich', pronounced 'trike' by Australian doctors and 'trick' by British ones) is, like almost all sexually transmitted infections, asymptomatic in the majority of humans that it infects – they simply don't know they've got it. Only a small proportion of people infected will exhibit any symptoms, and this is one of the reasons that the condition can become so common in a population: if people are unaware they are infected then they will not seek medical attention and treatment. However, when symptoms do occur, they are often quite troubling: women can develop a frothy and unpleasant smelling vaginal discharge, and men may have a discharge from the penis and pain when they urinate.

Unlike gonorrhoea and chlamydia, which are able to move up a woman's reproductive tract – from the cervix, into the uterus and through to the Fallopian tubes and into the pelvic cavity, where they cause pelvic inflammatory disease (PID) – T. vaginalis only likes to live in the vagina or the urethra. This means it rarely, if ever, results in the scarring of the Fallopian tubes and consequent infertility that is a feature of long-term PID. Nevertheless, trichomoniasis is important for two reasons: infection increases the risk of premature labour, and the inflammation of the vagina and urethra that it causes makes it easier to acquire and transmit HIV infection. It has been estimated that in populations where it is endemic, trichomoniasis could be responsible for as much as 20 per cent of the HIV infections that occur. These reproductive health and infectious interactions represent significant public health issues in populations where the disease is common. Unfortunately, instead of reducing the risk of premature labour, the treatment of trichomoniasis during pregnancy actually raises it slightly – an unexpected and disappointing finding. This is probably because women with no symptoms have not mounted much of an immune response to the organism: their immune systems have established a relationship of mutual acceptance with the parasite. When antibiotics are administered to kill the organism, the local immune response of the body to the now dead organisms produces inflammation in the vagina and cervix, which may trigger premature labour. This counter-intuitive finding doesn't mean that trichomoniasis should not be treated if symptoms become apparent – having it still increases the risk of premature labour in the women who haven't achieved an immunological détente with the organism.

The only way to reduce the premature labour associated directly with the bug or with its treatment, is to lower the prevalence of the disease in the general population so that women don't contract the infection in the first place.

Several years ago, one of our laboratory staff, a cytologist, asked me where trichomoniasis had gone. She had been examining Pap smears for more than 30 years and during the 1970s the parasite was a regular finding, but now she never saw it. This was also the experience of her cytologist colleagues, and none of them had an explanation for its disappearance. In fact, it was probably her own work which was largely responsible for the change: it is likely that doctors who got back positive trichomoniasis cytology reports after sending off patients' Pap smears, would have treated the women, and possibly the male partners as well. Although the Pap smear is not a very sensitive test for trichomoniasis – it only detects the disease 50 per cent of the time – because the majority of women have a Pap smear every two years since a co-ordinated program of screening for cervical cancer began in the early 1980s, most women with the infection would have been detected and treated eventually. When the male partners of the infected women were also treated this may have been enough to interrupt the transmission of the condition in the general population. (Although no vaccines are involved, this phenomenon is a variant of the herd immunity that we encountered in chapter 5.)

But it may have been the emergence and treatment of another condition that was the final nail in the lid of the parasite's tiny coffin. In the 1980s, doctors began to recognise a non-transmissible cause of vaginal discharge called bacterial vaginosis or BV *(see page 120)*. BV is treated with metronidazole, the same drug that is used to treat trichomoniasis. It is feasible that many women with asymptomatic trichomoniasis received treatment for it inadvertently when they presented to their doctor with symptomatic BV.

Metronidazole was invented by the French and was first used to treat trichomoniasis in 1959. Now off-patent and extremely cheap, the drug is best known as Flagyl, its original trade name. The drug soon made its way to the rest of Europe and to Australia, where its main use was for the treatment of anaerobic bacteria. Most people believe that you shouldn't drink alcohol when you are taking antibiotics. While some doctors may advise this as a punishment for contracting an STI in the first place, the truth is that a small amount of alcohol is unlikely to significantly interact with antibiotics and cause any side-effects. Except in the case of metronidazole. A small proportion of people who take metronidazole and drink alcohol become severely nauseated and vomit. The reaction is similar to that caused by the pill Antabuse (disulfiram), which was once widely used as an avoidance treatment for alcoholics. Antabuse blocks the action of alcohol dehydrogenase, which is the enzyme responsible for breaking down alcohol. Unfortunately the toxic metabolite which built up in the blood as a result could on rare occasions cause death when a patient fell off the wagon. Although the connection between metronidazole and such side-effects has been questioned recently, most authorities still recommend avoidance of the combination.

Metronidazole had a bad press in the USA because it was believed to be associated with birth defects when taken in pregnancy. These fears were unfounded, but as a result the drug was not widely used in the USA until the late 1980s, which could partly explain the relative persistence of trichomoniasis there compared to Europe and Australia.

A population under the radar

When I finished my infectious diseases training, trichomoniasis was a clinical curiosity – an exotic disease that older doctors remembered and younger ones read about in the STI textbooks.

A family doctor, or even a venereologist, working in a big city in the 1990s would probably never diagnose a case in a patient unless there was a history of overseas travel. When I moved to work in Darwin I did not have a sense of the significance of the disease or its local epidemiology until I read a paper published in the Australian journal, *Venereology*. A doctor trained in microbiology working in Alice Springs had, after obtaining permission from the local Aboriginal health centre and the regional ethics committee, examined the Pap smear records from the area and found that trichomoniasis was present in around 15 per cent of them. If the lack of sensitivity of the Pap smear was taken into account, the actual number of women infected would be about 30 per cent. When a disease has a rate this high it is sometimes referred to as hyper-endemic, yet the condition didn't appear on the diagnostic radar of the local clinicians, who would have been trained in places outside the Northern Territory, where the disease did not exist.

I remember being shocked by the findings. Trichomoniasis was not a notifiable disease and so the number of people infected was not available in any of the routine data collections. I was keen to know if the pathogen was as common in the Top End of the Territory as it was in central Australia, and if it was really important. I consulted with a microbiologist in Sydney. 'Never see it', he said. When I told him that up to 30 per cent of the Aboriginal female population in Alice Springs could have it, he told me that it must be 'normal flora' – in other words, a component of the myriad of harmless bugs that colonise a woman's vagina. When I mentioned the prevalence of the disease to one of the local doctors in Darwin she commented that 'something so common couldn't be a disease'.

I couldn't agree with either of my colleagues but wasn't quite sure how to prove otherwise. Then, late one afternoon, I received a fax from Kit Fairley in England.

A project is born

Kit and I had trained as registrars together at Fairfield hospital and he was currently in the UK, working as a post-doctoral fellow. His thesis had been on the epidemiology of the human papillomavirus, or HPV. Today it is accepted that HPV is the cause of cancer of the cervix (and there is mounting evidence that it causes a number of other cancers as well). In the early 1990s, however, the medical world was still trying to prove the relationship and to understand how the virus was spread.

HPV is a very common infection – in most societies the majority of women who are sexually active will become infected with at least one strain of the virus in their lifetime. That sex was involved in its transmission seemed a logical conclusion – but could it be spread in other ways? One of Kit's original research questions was whether or not virgins contracted HPV. This simple question was extremely difficult to answer – at the time there were no routine diagnostic tests available for HPV and the new PCR technology which could amplify miniscule bits of viral DNA was still just emerging as a powerful research tool (*see page 142*). Before he'd left for the UK, Kit had been working at the Royal Women's Hospital in Melbourne with Suzanne Garland and Sepehr Tabrizi, who had developed a method for detecting HPV in specimens from Pap smears. Since women who had never had sex did not have the test it was difficult to know how to collect samples from them for HPV testing.

Kit was describing the problem to his parents over dinner one night – believe me, medical families do this sort of thing – and his father, a renowned kidney specialist, said that the obvious solution would be to collect the women's used tampons and measure for any HPV DNA deposited on them. Kit took his father's idea and turned it into a technique for testing for HPV in women who had never had sex. Kit and his collaborators were soon able to show that none of the virgins that they tested had HPV.

When he moved to the UK to work on other things, Kit maintained his interest in HPV. He knew that I was involved in Aboriginal health, where STIs were a major public health issue. His fax asked if I could help him look at the epidemiology of HPV in the Northern Territory. I most certainly would, I wrote back, but only if we extended the range of the testing to include the STIs that were endemic in the population – chlamydia, gonorrhoea, and trichomoniasis. In the preceding few years, a number of laboratories had described PCR techniques for detecting these infections and the technical issues would be reasonably simple to solve. At the time, however, molecular biology was not routinely used for diagnosis – gonorrhoea could only be cultured in the traditional way, and chlamydia was detected using kits that were known to return both false negative and false positive results. No one had used the trichomoniasis PCR in any field studies up to this point; it would, therefore, be an exciting and important project. But, I thought, as I watched my reply to Kit stutter its way into the fax machine, I am going to have to convince people that using tampons for diagnosis is feasible in the Aboriginal population. That should be easy, I said, in an ironic aside to no one in particular.

Considering the harm that it is able to inflict upon the humans that it invades, the organism that causes gonorrhoea, *Neisseria gonorrhoeae*, is a sensitive little thing. It can't live very long outside its human host and it dies quickly if it is heated, cooled or dried. This constitutional frailty posed considerable problems to people trying to diagnose gonorrhoea in patients living in remote areas of Australia. If a nurse in a bush community saw a patient that she thought might have the disease, she would need to take a swab from the cervix in a woman, or the urethra in a man, and send it to the nearest laboratory. For the majority of clinics this would mean transport in a four-wheel-drive for hundreds of kilometres and, in some cases, a flight in a light plane. The specimen could take days to reach the laboratory and could be subjected to extreme heat in the process. The majority of specimens were degraded by the time they reached the laboratory and the bugs long dead. The new PCR techniques offered a solution. The DNA in the samples was theoretically much more stable than the living organisms themselves, and we hypothesised that specimens collected in the bush and which spent a long time in the back of a Landcruiser might still yield useful results using PCR for diagnosis. But we didn't know at the time if this was true.

Another barrier to diagnosing the condition in women was the need to obtain specimens from the cervix: in women, gonorrhoea doesn't live in the vagina itself but can only really survive in the cervix or urethra. To collect a swab from these sites you needed to perform a speculum examination – something which is intrusive, requires training and, of course, a willing patient. In places where the disease was extremely common this would mean that women required frequent speculum examinations, and it was believed by many health workers in the bush that this was turning people away from clinics. In theory, the exquisite sensitivity of the PCR technique could obviate the need for a speculum examination: only a very small amount of gonococcal DNA would be required for the assay and this could be obtained by taking a swab from anywhere in the vagina, or even at its outer reaches, the vulva. A sterile tampon straight out of its packaging could be used as a swab to collect the DNA from the vagina, and this simple procedure could be performed without the assistance of a nurse or Aboriginal health worker: for the first time testing could be, literally, in the hands of the patient herself.

I started to discuss the possibilities of using tampons for diagnosis with the local health workforce and enlisted the help of Barbara Paterson, then a doctor working in Darwin and later the Territory's chief health officer. She quickly saw the advantages of the approach but she knew that we would meet considerable resistance from colleagues. We soon found that the district medical officers, doctors who provided services to the regional health areas, were, to put it mildly, lukewarm about the proposal. 'Aboriginal women don't use tampons', one of them told me, 'and it wouldn't be culturally acceptable'. I put the idea to A. – an Aboriginal health worker who had recently commenced working in my clinic. She was a dynamic woman in her early 50s who looked a lot like Tina Turner. Her face dropped when I floated the proposal, which didn't fill me with confidence. However, after a night of reflection, she came to me and said that she thought it was a 'goer'. We were concerned about the comment that Aboriginal people in the bush didn't use tampons – the whole rationale for using them was that the sampling method would be a slight modification of something that women were already used to doing themselves dozens of times a year. Our fears quickly abated when Barbara and A. made a few phone calls to stores in remote communities and asked them if they stocked tampons and who bought them. The answer was yes, and they were sold by the hundreds of packets a month, mainly to Aboriginal women.

After a few months of intensive consultation with communities and health staff, we obtained ethics approval to undertake a formal study of the acceptability and utility of tampons for the diagnosis of STIs. To avoid having to use the word tampon, Barbara Paterson coined the term 'T-test' for the study.

Because this was clearly 'women's business' the responsibility for the operational aspects of the project was left up to A. and Barbara, who spent further time preparing the women and staff in remote communities. Everywhere they went they were met enthusiastically and once the study had begun A. received a number of calls from women in communities not included in it who had heard about the T-test and wanted to take part.

It was immediately apparent that the T-test was acceptable – the feedback we received from the women and the staff involved was invariably positive. The technology was innovative – this was the first time that such a comprehensive assessment of STIs in one patient had ever been undertaken anywhere in the world. But the results from the laboratory testing were shocking to say the least. We were detecting so much infection in the women who were volunteering for the study that we started to doubt the laboratory results – could it be true that so much disease existed in the communities? Were many of the results false positives? Sepehr Tabrizi double-checked the methods and went to great lengths in the laboratory to confirm that the results were true positives. In the end we were confident that the techniques gave an accurate result. We found that 42 per cent of the women had HPV, 25 per cent had trichomoniasis, 17 per cent had gonorrhoea and 11 per cent had chlamydia. Anyone working in the Northern Territory knew that STIs were an important public health issue, but we didn't know that things were this bad.

The T-test program was not confined to Aboriginal women – we were also testing non-Aboriginal women. Again, we found the approach acceptable to the participants and we identified some striking differences between the two groups. In the non-Aboriginal women, there were virtually no cases of trichomoniasis, gonorrhoea was rare and they had less than half the rate of chlamydia of their indigenous counterparts. This was not surprising to anyone working in the field but the next finding was: the non-Aboriginal women had slightly more HPV infection than the Aboriginal women. I was so fixated on the number of bacterial infections that we had identified in remote communities that I didn't appreciate the significance of this finding. But Kit in the UK did.

Changing the discourse

The fathers of mathematical modelling of infectious diseases, Roy Anderson and Bob May, showed in the 1980s that it is possible to plot the course of an STI epidemic if you can work out just three things: the probability that someone will catch the disease when they have sex; the time that the person remains infectious if they catch the disease; and the average number of partners that they have in a given time. Now, as they say, the devil is in the detail – it is incredibly difficult to accurately estimate each of these parameters, but knowing that this is all you have to consider allows you to break an epidemic into its component parts and consider, in a logical manner, the ways it could be controlled. For example, the amount of gonorrhoea in a population could be reduced by increasing the proportion of people wearing condoms during intercourse to reduce the likelihood of them coming into contact with the secretions of an infected partner. This seems obvious, and you don't need a mathematical model to tell you that condoms prevent infections. What the model does allow you to do, however, is calculate the proportion of people that need to wear condoms to control the epidemic. Models are about averages, not individuals, and they get a hard time from sectors of the medical profession; they are treated with healthy scepticism by some doctors and with cynicism by others. Doctors are mainly interested in the patient in front of them and they know that all generalisations are false.

Sometimes, however, a model provides an insight into a problem that may not be immediately obvious. For example, models tell us that the time it takes to locate and treat people with gonorrhoea can have a profound effect on the epidemic – possibly even more than promoting condom use. The effect that modification of one of the components of Anderson and May's STI equation will have depends on the biological properties of the disease being studied: what works for gonorrhoea may not work for HPV. For example, condoms may be less effective in the control of an HPV epidemic because the virus lesions can occur on parts of the genitalia where wearing a condom fails to provide a barrier.

Having seen the data that we were generating, Kit rang me

one morning in a state of some excitement. He told me to look at the HPV results.

'It is reasonable to assume', he said, 'that the duration of infectiousness and the risk of transmission of HPV is the same for both the Aboriginal and non-Aboriginal women in our study'.

'Sure.' I wasn't quite sure where he was going at this stage in the conversation.

'So if they are the same', he went on, 'then that only leaves the rate of partner change as the component of the equation that would be different between the groups'. But that led to a conclusion that was exactly the opposite of what most people would have expected, because our data supported the hypothesis that the non-Aboriginal women had *more* sexual partners over a defined period of time than the Aboriginal women.

'The samples are probably biased', I replied. The non-Aboriginal women that we tested were attending the urban clinics. They had self-selected themselves because they had symptoms or because they were worried that they had been involved in high-risk sexual behaviour. By contrast, the Aboriginal women from remote areas were more likely to have represented a random sample of the population.

'We would have selected a group of non-Aboriginal women who had a higher risk of HPV than the general population', I suggested.

'So why', Kit asked, 'if the non-Aboriginal women are at higher risk for infection, is there 100 times more trichomoniasis, 15 times more gonorrhoea and twice as much chlamydia in the Aboriginal women?' I couldn't answer that.

'Trichomoniasis, gonorrhoea and chlamydia are curable with simple antibiotic treatment, but HPV is an incurable virus. There is a difference in the STI rates because the Aboriginal women cannot get to, or they don't use, the services that could identify and treat their bacterial STIs.'

I didn't accept his explanation immediately – the major

reason being that I didn't want to admit that he had seen something so important and I had missed it – but by the next day I could see that he was right. While there was no question that sex was the means of transmission and that reducing the rate of partner change would have an effect on the amount of disease in the community, a more important determinant was the lack of availability of testing and treatment services for STIs in remote populations. This was something that we could influence more easily than the complex societal and cultural factors that determine sexual behaviour. More importantly, this could change the discourse from one of 'promiscuity' and 'sexual abstinence' to one that considered the physical constraints placed on service delivery in the bush.

(Since we did this work the role that sexual networks play in the development of STI epidemics has become clearer and adds a further degree of complexity to the modelling. It seems that if a population has a proportion of people who have more than one partner at the same time, called concurrency, this may increase the level of infection in the community more than if they have only one partner at a time, called serial monogamy. The total number of partners in a year might be the same in both populations, but the group who have more concurrent partners will have a bigger epidemic. This offers another insight into the drivers of the epidemic and provides new options for health promotion.)

I had been the target of criticism from many quarters because I was prepared to talk publicly about STIs in Aboriginal populations. Some government doctors thought that I was pushing a professional barrow to highlight my own interests. Some doctors in the community questioned the importance of STIs as a public health issue in the first place, and others felt that the information brought to light by the study only added to the stigma that was already a daily part of Aboriginal people's lives. Publication of our data would only feed redneck stereotypes, they said – and to a certain extent they could have been right. However, I believed that unless we brought the issues into the open there would be no hope of making any progress. Indeed, I had gained the impression from my clinical work that many Aboriginal health workers themselves believed that the differential in STI rates was related to sexual rather than to medical factors: we now had data and a plausible hypothesis that could change the way people in communities and in government could think about the 'STI problem'.

Our findings were published in the *Journal of the American Medical Association* (JAMA). Dissemination of information in the peer-reviewed medical literature is the essential first step in changing practice – it establishes the academic credentials of the work, but it is not enough in itself. Hardly anybody in Australia has ever read our JAMA paper. The next step had to be to influence the thinking of the medical profession, the opinion leaders in the community, and, most importantly, the people who held the funding purse-strings. Fortunately there were people working in the Office of Aboriginal and Torres Strait Islander Health (OATSIH) in the Commonwealth health department who were receptive to our ideas. They were in the late stages of finalising the first National Indigenous Australians' Sexual Health Strategy (NIASHS) and I later learnt that our findings were to be influential in their deliberations.

Tactical wins and strategic losses

It was apparent that the control of STIs in remote communities would require not just an investment of money but a change in the way the medical workforce thought about them. At the time, screening was a dirty word in many Aboriginal health circles. Debates, sometimes unpleasant, had raged at scientific meetings in the Northern Territory, where those who proposed screening in any shape or form were accused of being paternalistic and discriminatory. A commonly heard put-down was that screening was a 'sheep dip' approach. One edition of the Central Australian Rural Practitioners Association's newsletter in the early 1990s had published a series of criticisms of a discussion paper written by the director of the Menzies School of Health Research, John Mathews. In it he proposed that some infectious diseases that were endemic in Aboriginal communities could be controlled through a program of screening and treatment. Some of the responses from the local practitioners argued against the practice on scientific grounds, but others seemed to be ideologically opposed, equating it with the mission days of lining people up and telling them what to do. The front cover of the CARPA newsletter showed a picture of a scientist in a white coat looking down a microscope. A thought bubble read: 'Looks like it's sheep dip then … '

The experience of Aboriginal people with health systems had made them justifiably suspicious of medical interventions, and the word screening evoked powerful anamnestic responses. But we argued that a consultative and respectful approach to screening was possible, and OATSIH produced a strategy document that included an endorsement of screening and recommended that funds be made available for the new PCR technology, which at the time was not on the Medicare Benefit Schedule.

The best way to get people to your table is to put money on it, and so the offer of funding for screening activities was a powerful spur to action. Programs began outside the Northern Territory, and it was soon apparent that STIs were also hyperendemic in other parts of remote Australia. We had been just ahead of the technological wave: soon commercial kits for the detection of chlamydia and gonorrhoea were released, though none for trichomoniasis (which remains the case, with practitioners reliant on in-house kits produced by local laboratories). We learnt too that we didn't have to continue with the T-test – the usual swabs available for other microbiological testing would do almost as good a job. This opened up diagnostic testing to laboratories across the country that didn't have experience with the T-test. By the millennium the word screening no longer rankled. The tools to allow easy testing were in place, there was a willingness to do it, and programs were running. Screening would be shown to be an acceptable public health strategy wherever it was conducted with proper attention to the rights and wishes of the local communities and individual patients. In central Australia, one network of remote health clinics run by the Nganampa Health Service demonstrated sustained reductions in syphilis, chlamydia and gonorrhoea by the adoption of regular screening programs, and these results were replicated by health services elsewhere in the country. In the Northern Territory, outcomes were less positive: although one Top End community was able to achieve reduced rates of chlamydia, in most places the STI infection figures did not show much change.

Comprehensive screening is time-consuming, costly and places a considerable burden on local health service staff. The competing demands of other health issues can lower the priority given to STI programs. As a result, the in-principle adoption of screening has not resulted in a major change in the overall prevalence of most STIs in remote Australia. While there have been a number of important successes *(see chapter 11)*, the number of Aboriginal patients with chlamydia and gonorrhoea has increased over the past ten years, and the difference between the rates in the Aboriginal and the non-Aboriginal populations remains stark.

Rumblings that screening was a waste of time started to be heard in Aboriginal health circles and people began to suggest that the idea itself was flawed. But it was not screening per se that was the problem, rather it was the failure to properly implement the part of the program that really makes the difference – the treatment bit.

Our modelling had shown that to halve the prevalence of a disease as common and as easily transmitted as trichomoniasis it would be necessary to screen 50 per cent of the at-risk population every six months. The lack of adequate funding and staff shortages meant that this was beyond the capacity of the health services in remote communities. It was time to think differently about STI control in the bush – again.

13

Let's *not* talk about sex

Chlamydia trachomatis – an intracellular sexually transmitted
bacterium. Because it cannot be grown in routine culture media
C. trachomatis was only fully characterised as a human pathogen
in the 1960s. Most people with the bacterium are unaware that
they are infected and a proportion of women develop pelvic
inflammatory disease and tubal scarring that may lead to ectopic
pregnancy and tubal factor infertility. The organism is also
the cause of the eye disease trachoma, which is not sexually
transmitted.

'My brain? That's my second favorite organ.' (Woody Allen,
1935–)

When I first moved to my current hospital it took me several
months to convince the surgeon administrator who controlled
outpatients that I needed a clinic space to see my patients with
infectious diseases. For a month I had been treating a gentle
woman in her 70s in hospital for an MRSA infection in her knee.
It had been difficult to manage – she had become allergic to the
antibiotics I was using and I had to change her to a second-line
agent that was causing some quite unpleasant side-effects. When
she was finally able to take oral antibiotics and could be sent
home, I had nowhere to review her in outpatients. My main job

at the time was as director of the sexual health centre, so while the silly fight about clinic space was going on, I had to see my general infectious diseases patients in the centre as well.

People who haven't ever attended a sexual health centre might be surprised to learn that the posters on the wall of the waiting room are usually a little more ... shall I say, interesting than the ones that may be posted in the average GP's clinic. The magazines, too, target a different demographic, and the educational video which played on our small TV was not alerting our patients to the connection between a poor diet and diabetes, but rather to the potential perils of a somewhat more private activity.

My patient was accompanied to the clinic by her husband, a proper and well-connected man who had supervised my treatment of his wife in the same way that he would have supervised a contract during his working life.

I couldn't have deliberately arranged the composition of the other patients in the waiting room that day to better reflect the diversity of our clientele. Two girls, still in their school uniforms, sat sullenly in one corner, a middle-aged man with a handlebar moustache and leather pants sat in another, a woman, slightly over-dressed for a Monday morning but underdressed in other ways, stood reading one of the posters. As I led this mannerly couple down the corridor to my room I apologised that they had to be seen in the sexual health centre. By the time they were sitting next to my desk, they were both wearing broad grins.

'You don't have to apologise', said the husband. 'We told all our friends that we were coming here today to see you. It's already done wonders for our reputation at the bridge club.'

I have always tried to anticipate and accommodate the sensitivities of my patients, but even for someone like me, who has spent a considerable proportion of his professional life talking about sex, the way that people respond to these most private matters can be very difficult to predict.

What, where, who and how often?

Being originally, and probably essentially, an infectious diseases doctor, many of my venereologist colleagues are a bit suspicious of my attitude towards sex. It is not that I lack interest – domestically, at least – but from a professional perspective I have always been more focused on germs than on sex. Nevertheless, an understanding of the range of sexual behaviour in a population at a particular time is essential: it helps us to know which infections people are at risk of catching. For example, consider the current vogue among young people for oral sex: it carries the risk of transmitting or catching genital herpes, syphilis and gonorrhoea, but is very unlikely to lead to the transmission of HIV. Conversely, receptive anal sex carries a very high risk of transmission of HIV, insertive anal sex, a little less risk. Vaginal intercourse carries a low risk of HIV, but chlamydia and HPV are easily transmitted this way. Condom use is highly protective against some STIs but not others. There is no medical specialty that offers a better marriage of epidemiology and clinical medicine than sexual health. If, with regard to a particular sexually transmitted infection, you know what people are doing, where they are doing it, who they are doing it with and how often – that is, you understand its epidemiology – then you are equipped with the knowledge that will allow you to devise a way of controlling that infection. But since STIs usually don't betray themselves by symptoms in the people they infect, how might doctors go about obtaining such information from patients, who usually come to see them over an unrelated health matter? The answer is to encourage greater uptake of the procedure that by definition identifies an illness or condition in a person who has no idea that they may have it – screening. It is a public health activity based on the inescapably paternalistic premise that we know something about you that you don't know – which brings us to chlamydia.

Top of the communicable diseases pops

We know from studies that between 5 and 6 per cent of Australian women between the ages of 20 and 25 have chlamydia, but 80 per cent of these women will be unaware that they are infected because they do not have any recognisable symptoms. Chlamydia is a rather effete organism – it can't be grown on the agar plates that you find in a microbiology laboratory because it requires human cells to complete its life cycle. This technical problem meant that *Chlamydia trachomatis* was not fully identified as a pathogen until the 1960s, and the disease it caused was only easily diagnosed in the 1980s. For this reason the bug was not embedded in the sexual folklore of previous generations in the same way as gonorrhoea and syphilis. It has taken a decade of health promotion to raise awareness of the pathogen's 'brand'.

C. trachomatis lives in the urethra of men and women, and on the female cervix. Usually it just sits and waits for an opportunity to transfer itself to another host and fulfill its mindless evolutionary destiny by reproducing. Sometimes, however, the host produces a vigorous immune response to the bacterium, which causes inflammation and, in turn, symptoms. While the young man with gonococcal urethritis may complain of 'pissing razorblades', chlamydial urethritis is usually milder – perhaps 'pissing slightly blunted kitchen knives' would be the parallel analogy. Women usually have no idea they are infected: chlamydia doesn't produce a vaginal discharge and cervical infection is usually 'silent', although there may be subtle clues, such as bleeding after intercourse or mid-cycle 'spotting'. The real problem with chlamydia is that in a proportion of infections on the cervix, the microbe travels up through the uterus and into the Fallopian tubes. If this happens, the tubes become inflamed and can cause local symptoms such as pain during intercourse and lower abdominal pain – so-called pelvic inflammatory disease, although this can also be caused by gonorrhoea and several non-sexually transmitted bacterial infections. A sub-set of these women will develop scarring of the Fallopian tubes, and this results in a high risk of infertility and ectopic pregnancy (where the embryo is implanted in the tube instead of the uterus). Complications in men are less common, but include painful inflammation of the testes and epididymis (the tubular vessel attached to the testes, where sperm are stored). Only very rarely does this lead to male infertility, and it is the potential reproductive complications in women that make chlamydial infection a public health problem. In 2009 there were over 62 000 chlamydia infections notified in Australia, making it easily the top of the communicable diseases pops.

A test just waiting to happen

A sophisticated health system has a responsibility to alert women to these facts and establish a program to protect their reproductive futures. If chlamydia is mainly a silent or asymptomatic infection, what will facilitate screening? The answer is public awareness of the need for testing, coupled with a receptive medical workforce. (I have called this approach 'bottom up, top down', although it doesn't quite sound right in this context.) We have a wonderful example of a program that has successfully achieved this in Australia: the co-ordinated cervical cancer screening program – usually known as the Pap smear program – which has substantially reduced the death rate from cervical cancer over the past 25 years. Until recently, women didn't know that cervical cancer was caused by a sexually transmitted infection – the human papillomavirus (HPV). Asking for a Pap smear, or accepting the offer from your doctor, was in no way associated with any sense of stigma, and a middle-class married matron from a leafy suburb could just as happily go in for her screening as a grunge band groupie.

But chlamydia is different: it has always been framed as a sexually transmitted infection and no matter how hard we try to de-stigmatise it, the sex word gets in the way. A constant finding of surveys about barriers to screening for chlamydia in general practice is that doctors have difficulty discussing sexual matters with patients unless it is the patient who raises the subject. The logical solution proffered from some parts of the sexual health community is that training for doctors needs to be improved so that they can become more proficient at taking what is known as a sexual history. Logical, but is it right?

I spend a lot of time with my students and junior doctors teaching them the importance of taking a sexual history. In fact there is probably more sexual health built into our curriculum than that of any other medical school in the country. We teach our students that a patient with symptoms that are suggestive of an STI who makes a conscious decision to attend a sexual health centre or GP's surgery to seek help for those symptoms will not be shocked if the doctor asks about intimate matters relating to their sex life. And we teach them to be competent and comfortable in asking those questions. In addition, we point out the importance of taking a sexual history from all patients with a serious illness, because knowing about this usually hidden facet of a person's life is essential in many different clinical con-texts: a young man presenting to hospital with a high fever after returning from Bangkok, where he had sex with a local women in a nightclub, could have HIV infection; an infected knee joint in a Rugby player returning from the end-of-year trip to the Philip-pines could be gonorrhoea; the whole body rash of the married businessman who spent a night in a San Francisco bath-house could be syphilis. A few tactfully put questions can pave the way for the appropriate tests.

But what about when a 19-year-old male basket-baller arrives in a GP's surgery with a strained knee ligament: will the doctor take a sexual history and offer a chlamydia test while he is applying the bandage? Or when a 24-year-old woman goes to her doctor with hay fever: should she receive a chlamydia screening test plus a prescription for a nasal spray? In an ideal world the answer is yes, but in the real world this just doesn't happen in most general practice encounters.

Family doctors are always being asked to screen for something – blood pressure, diabetes, cholesterol, depression and so on. The health promotion that supports these diseases is often heavily backed by the pharmaceutical industry, and so the doctor and the patient have the messages constantly reinforced in their mind. Industry does spend money on the marketing of some products related to sex – drugs such as Viagra are heavily promoted in the medical press and advertisements for antiviral drugs for genital herpes even appear in the mainstream media. But, as the drug company rep character played by Jake Gyllenhal in the film *Love and other drugs* found out, the potential earnings from the treatment of chlamydia are chicken feed compared to the billions that pills for erectile dysfunction and depression can generate. There is little commercial reason, therefore, for GPs and their patients to be primed to talk about chlamydia treatment.

So here is my suggestion: when it comes to chlamydia screening, let's *not* talk about sex. We know who is at the greatest risk of chlamydia in the general Australian population – sexually active people between the ages of 15 and 29. We could introduce a system that routinely offers this group a chlamydia test that depends solely on their age. No need to ask the sex questions of 'who', 'how many', or 'how often'. No room for excuses for inaction that include not knowing how to take a 'proper' sexual history, or not having the time to take one.

In 2006 we conducted a trial that showed we could double the rate of screening for chlamydia that occurred in general practice by simply suggesting to GPs that they offered a chlamydia test to patients at the same time as they were having a Pap test.

Since about 50 per cent of women between the ages of 20 and 29 have a Pap test every two years this strategy has the potential to screen half the population of women for chlamydia in this age range every two years. I am not saying that you won't have to ultimately talk about sex to the women who test positive (about six in every 100 screened) but that a female patient's decision about testing should not be contingent on such a discussion. Our study showed that this approach was highly acceptable to both the doctors and women sampled, and that it didn't significantly prolong consultations. Whenever I discuss this idea with non-medical groups or journalists they look at me as if to say, 'you mean this isn't already happening?' Yet there has been enormous resistance from some quarters of the medical profession to the idea of this combination of testing. Critics argue that it only targets women in one age group and doesn't apply to men. True. However, the sexual partners of women found to be infected are tested and treated as part of the contact-tracing that follows. Other critics worry that participation in the Pap program could fall if it was 'contaminated' by the realisation that testing for a sexually transmitted infection formed part of it. I think that this is a little patronising towards young women in the 21st century, and it ignores our empiric evidence to the contrary. Others argue that the advent of the HPV vaccine and the likely changes to the schedule for Pap smears in the next few years (the recommended interval between tests may be extended to three years from the current two) reduce the value of combined testing. This is a reasonable comment, but while we wait for these changes to be made it would seem logical to extend the current program to include screening for chlamydia. It is now four years since our original study, and the Pap screening protocols in Australia haven't changed yet.

A monetary incentive works wonders

The Pap/chlamydia test is just part of a wider solution. Other strategies are needed to encourage women under 20 years old to be screened. In 2008 we conducted a study which paid people to have a chlamydia test. For more than ten years in Australia we have provided doctors with incentives to provide particular services to their patients. The Commonwealth Department of Health and Ageing offers 13 different Practice Incentive Payments to encourage doctors to offer, among other things, cervical screening, domestic violence assessment and diabetes treatment. We proposed that it should be possible to apply these simple economics to the demand side of the equation.

Traditional STI health promotion can mean health workers spending weeks and months in schools, universities, TAFE campuses, and at sports and music events telling young people that they should get a chlamydia test, that what they don't know *can* hurt them, that they need to protect their future fertility – all true and honourable things. Hardly any of their audience take any notice and get tested, though. We applied this approach for six months and were delighted to obtain 627 specimens. When we trialled a $10 cash incentive payment, however, we received 392 specimens in three days. Money talks to young people, and, most important of all, we saw twice as many men as women participate in the trial – the exact opposite of the ratio observed in every other screening setting.

Many professionals involved in health promotion find this approach very challenging and some are outright opposed to the use of cash incentives for anyone but the providers of the service – despite their clear effectiveness and potential to allow the staff involved in screening to offer the program in multiple sites because of the improved ratio of staff hours required to number of tests obtained.

The holy grail of chlamydia control is a government-funded,

co-ordinated program that would automatically invite young people to be screened and then send them reminders for follow-up screening every one or two years. Governments are wary of funding such a program because of the cost (cervical cancer screening costs more than $150 million annually). But one thing that is often forgotten is that chlamydia is an infection, not a chronic disease or cancer. An intensive campaign run over five or ten years could reduce the prevalence of chlamydia to a point where a general campaign would no longer be necessary. This happened in the case of TB after the mass screening programs of the 1950s and 60s. I am sure that we can achieve the same sort of decline where chlamydia is concerned.

Paradoxes and proposals

I am aware of the irony that, having spent a large part of my career trying to get people involved in Aboriginal health to talk more openly about sexual health, I should now be promoting the idea that we actually downplay cause and effect in the case of chlamydia. And if what I proposed about screening in the preceding section is controversial to mainstream medical opinion, then my ideas about Aboriginal health will cause, to put it mildly, a degree of disquiet. But it is in this sphere that I believe it is even more important to consider new strategies to lower the rates of sexually transmitted infections, because the approaches tried so far have simply not worked.

Consider the following paradox. As well as causing chlamydia, *C. trachomatis* is the cause of the eye disease trachoma. Both are prevalent in the Aboriginal population, yet the approach to these two diseases is very different. It has been suggested that Australia may become the last country in the world to have endemic trachoma – the disease may be eliminated in the developing world before it is finally controlled in the Aboriginal population.

Trachoma is a disease of poverty and lack of access to clean water. It affects children and young adults and, over many years, causes scarring of the eyelids that can ultimately progress to blindness. It is relatively easy to diagnose and, in its early stages, easy to treat. The World Health Organization recommends that if 10 per cent of a population are found to have trachoma then every child in that population, and every adult in the household of infected children, should receive a single oral dose of the long-acting antibiotic, azithromycin. This mass treatment approach has been shown to be effective in the sustained control of trachoma in countries in Africa with limited health infrastructures. A modification of this community antibiotic treatment approach has been recommended in Australia.

Genital chlamydia is also endemic in many remote Aboriginal populations. In some places around 10 per cent or more of the population are infected. This is at least three to four times higher than the prevalence of the infection in the rest of Australia. Yet to institute the same sort of mass treatment for genital chlamydia that is recommended for the control of trachoma is, in most quarters, unthinkable. Here are two diseases with similar behaviours – silent, slow to cause serious problems, disproportionately affecting the same group in the population, and with the same treatment options, but because one is an STI and the other is not, totally different approaches to their control are followed.

Chlamydia is afforded a special status in the public health sector because it is sexually transmitted. Many people believe that it would be wrong to treat it in the same way as trachoma, because this would not be 'holistic': we would be ignoring the complexities of the social setting that has led to the disease becoming endemic in the first place. I am not advocating that we ignore the social determinants of disease – far from it. The most important way to improve the health of a population is to ensure that its members are housed and have clean water and sanitation, and that through education they have employment opportunities and develop a sense of control over their destiny. But these are things that will take a generation to implement. Meanwhile, the present cohort of young people will suffer the consequences of the STIs they contract today unless something is done now – albeit as a stop-gap measure, and one which would need to be modified as the prevalence of disease falls.

When a vaccine is available for the control of an infection the health system will spend millions of dollars to ensure that the people who need the vaccine receive it. The initial HPV vaccine roll-out to all young Australian women cost more than $250 million – to protect them from an important, life-threatening, but, it has to be remembered, relatively rare cancer. I have no quarrel with this – in fact I was a strong advocate of the program as it was being considered for funding. However, if it is acceptable to offer vaccination to the entire female population to protect a small proportion from the serious consequences of HPV infection, why are we not willing to treat with antibiotics a population in which 10 per cent is infected with chlamydia and up to 25 per cent will have either chlamydia, gonorrhoea or trichomoniasis? It is true that antibiotics, unlike vaccines, do not induce immunity and have the potential to 'breed' resistant organisms, but – and this is a big 'but' – when STI infections have reached a prevalence where a quarter of the population is infected and there are no vaccines (HPV and hepatitis B are the only STI agents for which vaccines have been developed) one option is to treat all the people in that population. The screen-and-treat approach which we promoted heavily in the 1990s will only work when you can guarantee that the time between screening and treatment is short and you can reach enough of the potentially infected population.

There is an important concept in STI practice which contends that 20 per cent of the population are usually responsible for 80 per cent of infection – we call the 20 per cent a core group, and they are often the hardest group to reach. They may be young and reckless, alcoholic or using other drugs, they may have mental illness and lead chaotic lives. In this group a program that is only able to provide treatment a week after screening is unlikely to work because the chances of finding those whose tests return positive is low. Identifying those at high risk of infection, testing them, and then treating on the spot (before the result of the test is available) is, I believe, a legitimate approach. Kath Fethers and I proposed this in the *Medical Journal of Australia* in 2008, and the idea was not at all popular. We were criticised for taking a disease-focused approach that did not deal with the underlying social problems that resulted in such high levels of disease. Furthermore, in the context of STIs doctors seem wedded to idea that their patients must have tested positive before they can treat them. But doctors treat people with other infections all the time without having a firm microbiological diagnosis. It is generally acceptable to give what is known as empiric treatment for many collections of symptoms and clinical signs. For example, children in Top End communities are routinely de-wormed with antibiotics without proof that they are actually infected. All medications carry risks of adverse reactions – practise long enough and every doctor will see them for themselves – but we will usually treat straight away when the risk-to-benefit ratio tips in favour of benefit.

If you look outside the infectious diseases world, you will find that doctors are more than happy to give 'well' people drugs that they have to take not just once but every day. For example, patients with a cholesterol reading just above the normal limit have a slightly increased risk of having a heart attack and they, and their doctors, are very comfortable with the idea of life-long cholesterol-lowering therapy. It is only when you multiply the small benefit of the medication for the individual patient by the size of the whole population that it translates into a big public health effect. So I am disappointed that people cannot see that for a particular population with a terrible burden of sexually transmitted infections it would be justifiable to consider implementing a program that treated as many of the sexually active population as possible to reduce the amount of disease present. Under such a regimen of treatment, as the proportion of people with the diseases fell to a level approaching the mainstream, it would be logical to return to treating just those diagnosed with the disease. I know that people are worried that targeting specific diseases will be a distraction – that other elements of community development and public health will be neglected. This *could* happen but it is most certainly not the intention of the approach I am proposing. It *is* possible to walk and chew gum at the same time in public health.

I published the first detailed statistics about the profile of STIs in the Northern Territory in 1993. Eighteen years later, with the notable exceptions of a single disease (donovanosis) and a decline in the rates of STIs in several discrete communities, the number of Aboriginal people living in remote areas who contract a treatable STI each year had more than doubled. Business as usual will not do and there is a desperate need to carefully investigate and evaluate new ways of working. There is no harm in encouraging patients and health practitioners to talk openly about sex, but we must recognise that our in-built reluctance to do so can get in the way of devising effective treatment policies. However, if a barrier to a successful program is related to deeply-seated beliefs or to human nature itself, it will be easier, and more effective, to change what we do rather than who we are.

14

The Yellow Pages

There are six pathogens that are known as 'hepatitis viruses' and at a molecular level they are as different from one another as viruses can be; it is only their common ability to infect liver cells that binds them together as a group. Hepatitis B and C are linked by their means of transmission (blood-borne) and their potential to cause long-term, severe liver damage. Hepatitis A and E are transmitted through contaminated water and in faeces but don't cause long-term liver disease. Disease caused by hepatitis viruses is one of the most important contemporary public health problems facing both the developing and developed world.

'I wonder if illiterate people get the full effect of alphabet soup?'
(Jerry Seinfeld, 1954–)

My brother-in-law had been a patient in Fairfield Infectious Diseases Hospital in 1958. He had been a little unwell for a few days before his mother noticed that his eyes were yellow. She realised that he had 'yellow jaundice' and took him to their doctor. The GP diagnosed infectious hepatitis (inflammation of the liver) and sent the boy straight to the hospital. He had very few memories of his time there, and when I was working at the hospital in the 1980s he asked me to see if his medical record still existed.

As this was a hospital that stored blood from every single patient who came through the front gates, I wasn't surprised when the records clerk handed me a thin file. The entry notes were written in a beautiful copperplate – in fountain pen, of course – but there wasn't much to go on. There was a cursory admission note written by the resident: '8 year old boy with infectious hepatitis, anorectic one week, deeply jaundiced, pale stools. Tender in RUQ. Admit. Isolate. Observe'. The daily entries from the nursing staff were terse. One read: 'Ate breakfast. Vomited. Naughty boy'. The following day's note was even briefer: 'Better. Naughty boy'. The next few days' entries were similar, until the final entry of just four words, the first three underlined: 'Very naughty boy. Discharge'.

I never learnt what my brother-in-law did to incur the documented displeasure of the nursing staff. I remember his father telling me that one day his son had pushed a berry from a crab apple tree so far up his nose that he had to have it removed under anaesthetic. No one in the family doubted that he had annoyed the nursing staff.

Today a patient like that would be managed at home, but in the 1950s most people with an infectious disease were quarantined. Although it had not yet been identified, it was known that hepatitis was caused by a virus, not a bacterium, and so there was no place for penicillin or any of the other antibiotics that were rapidly appearing on the market. Admit. Isolate, Observe. In a time when people were frightened of Reds Under the Bed, many doctors would write COMI in the notes as an ironic instruction to the nurses (Careful Observation, Masterful Inactivity).

The paradox of changing sanitation

There are five hepatitis viruses with important repercussions for human health and, at a molecular level, they are as different from one other as viruses can be – the only thing that binds them together is their ability to damage the liver of the people that they infect.

My future brother-in-law had contracted what is now known as hepatitis A. The lay term yellow jaundice was not only tauto-logical but non-specific: jaundice is derived from the Old French word 'jaunice', which translates as 'yellowness', and is a symptom of many things other than an infection – gall stones and cancer of the pancreas to name just two. It was in 1973 that the virus was isolated and named logically, if a little unimaginatively, hep-atitis A. The pathogen is transmitted by what is quaintly referred to as the faecal-oral route; in other words the virus is excreted in the infected person's stool and finds its way to someone else's mouth via contaminated hands or food. It would make sense then that this was a disease of poor hygiene and sanitation, and that 'clean-living people', as my mother would call them, would be able to avoid the disease. But here is another of the fascinating paradoxes of infectious diseases: for a period of time societies moving from poor to good sanitation infrastructure are likely to experience more hepatitis A than a society without clean water supplies and proper sewers. How can this be?

When humans started living in close proximity to each other in towns and cities they were sharing more than a common purpose – they began to share each others' germs as well. In countries where sanitation is poor the water supply is routinely contaminated with faeces and so the majority of the population is exposed to hepatitis A in childhood – along with countless other bugs.

When children younger than five are infected with hepatitis A the disease is usually trivial and jaundice is uncommon. Infec-tion in childhood leads to lifelong immunity, and so the disease is rare in adults who grew up in places with poor sanitation. Epi-demiologists call this type of hepatitis A infection pattern A. As countries move from developing to developed they improve their plumbing. During the transition, pattern B infections occur: childhood infection becomes less common, so an increasing number of reach adulthood with no immunity to hepatitis A. The virus is still in circulation though, because the improvements in sanitation occur piecemeal, and so localised outbreaks of infection are common. Melbourne in the 1960s was such a city in transition – there were still many suburbs that did not have sewer systems. In the new 'War-Service Homes' suburb of Ashwood we had a septic tank in our back yard that I had to pump out by hand every week. Some households were still visited by the 'night cart man' (*see chapter 5*), who emptied the family drum of excreta each day. The hepatitis virus may have been in retreat but it was still in circulation in some parts of the city. Herd immunity waned, and so instead of being a silent infection of childhood, hepatitis A became for a while a very visible epidemic of older children and adolescents – a perverse effect of the long-awaited introduction of the city's sewage system. (Other bacteria transmitted through poor sanitation – for example typhoid, salmonella and shigella – are not childhood illnesses that produce lifelong immunity, so the arrival of the sewage system was an instant public health triumph for the prevention of these infections.)

Champagne doesn't give immunity

Illnesses that are meant to occur in childhood can cause very severe disease in adults. Hepatitis A is a good example of this. Instead of being a brief, and usually unrecognised illness, hepatitis A among a minority of adult sufferers can be prolonged and debilitating, and very occasionally (less than 1 per cent of cases) it causes liver failure and death. If you grew up in a country with longstanding good sanitation and visit the developing world, you are unlikely to have immunity and are at risk of contracting the disease. This is pattern C infection.

By 1980, the incidence of hepatitis A in Australia in those under 50 had declined dramatically, but if you were over 50 you were almost certain to have antibodies against it, thanks to infection while young. Now that almost all suburban Australia is sewered, the chance of encountering hepatitis A is extremely low, and the only protection available to an individual travelling to a country where the virus is still circulating is to get vaccinated before going. However, occasional outbreaks of hepatitis A still occur where there is sharing of faecal material – parliaments have, thus far, been spared, but childcare centres, schools and houses for the intellectually handicapped can be places of transmission. Gay men are at high risk through sexual activity, and a significant proportion will have naturally-acquired immunity. All of which, along with foreign travel, raises the little appreciated question of hand-washing after going to a toilet.

You can't get sick by infecting yourself with a bacterium or virus that is already in your own bowel, but you can make someone else sick by transmitting that pathogen to them. Hand-washing after ablutions is therefore an altruistic act – it lowers the risk of someone catching an illness from you. Of course this doesn't hold true if you touch a toilet seat, cistern button or tap that's been contaminated by an infected person: in this case hand-washing may be the way that you come in contact with the germs that you are trying to avoid passing on. Women have a harder job avoiding contamination in a toilet than men, who most frequently only use it for micturition – urine is usually sterile and poses no risk to another individual. Therefore, the socially unacceptable practice of not washing your hands after passing urine in a public toilet may be the more hygienic approach for a male. For women, who have to touch a seat and use toilet paper, the personal risk-to-benefit ratio favours hand-washing.

Occasional outbreaks of hepatitis A are associated with food-poisoning – in 1997 an epidemic occurred when an oyster farm on the Mid-North Coast of New South Wales was contaminated by sewage outfall. Over 400 people were infected and one elderly main died of acute liver failure. One of my colleagues refuses to eat oysters because he doesn't trust an animal which gets its nutrients by filtering hundreds of litres of potentially polluted seawater each day. 'Oysters kill Patrick', is one of his common warnings to seafood-loving friends.

The vaccine for hepatitis A was a relative latecomer – it wasn't released until 1993, after being developed in the USA – but it has a strong link to Australia. The vaccine is derived from a strain of the virus which was isolated from a Melbourne man who was a patient at Fairfield Hospital in the 1960s. For some reason this particular strain could be grown well in the laboratory and was suitable for the experiments needed to develop the vaccine. In a much more relaxed age of international air travel and quarantine regulation, Ian Gust, while director of the laboratory at Fairfield, carried vials of the virus to the USA in his luggage. Complete protection against hepatitis A is now possible. The problem is that the vaccine is expensive, and because the risk of hepatitis A is so low in developed countries, it is not cost-effective to include it on the childhood immunisation schedule. The vaccine is therefore targeted at people considered to be at high risk of infection – for example, healthcare and childcare workers, practising homosexual men and travellers to countries where the disease is endemic.

Some in these target groups ignore the advice. Last year a 40-year-old patient of mine had his honeymoon in Fiji and decided to use the $140 he would have spent on the vaccine to buy French champagne instead. He developed one of the worst cases of hepatitis A I had seen in years and it was three months of misery before he started to feel even half-normal.

The next letter's a bigger number

While most mothers in Melbourne in the 1960s would have had personal contact with infectious hepatitis, only a few would have encountered its nearest cousin, alphabetically speaking, 'transfusion hepatitis' – or, as it became officially known, hepatitis B. This virus infected a small proportion of people who had received blood transfusions or blood products, and it was starting to appear in the growing number of injecting drug users. It had been long established that the two types of hepatitis behaved very differently: hepatitis A or infectious hepatitis had an incubation period of between two and six weeks, while it took from six weeks to six months for the symptoms of hepatitis B or transfusion hepatitis to appear after the initial exposure. If you recovered from hepatitis A then that was the end of the matter – there were no long-term complications. Hepatitis B, however, could lead to long-term infection and, eventually, cirrhosis (or scarring) of the liver, liver failure and liver cancer.

The hepatitis B virus was identified in 1970, three years before hepatitis A. It soon became apparent that hepatitis B could be transmitted from an infected mother to her newborn and that it was endemic in Asia, parts of Africa and among Australia's Aboriginal population. (Indeed, in 1963 one of the proteins found in what would subsequently be called the hepatitis B virus was known as 'Australia antigen' because it was derived from a blood sample collected from a Western Australian Aboriginal.) The virus could be spread sexually and through contaminated hypodermic needles. Most people who acquire hepatitis B clear it from their system and are then immune to subsequent infection for life. However, around 5 per cent of those who acquire it as adults continue to carry the virus in their blood, and these people can transmit the infection to others. Infected newborns are almost certain to carry the infection throughout their life. For those unlucky enough to become chronically infected, between

15 and 25 per cent will develop cirrhosis or cancer of the liver.

Because of its long-term effects on the liver, hepatitis B is a far more serious infection than hepatitis A. The World Health Organization estimates that two billion people have been infected with hepatitis B and that 350 million remain chronically infected – the majority of these infections occur in China. Since the hepatitis B vaccine was released in 1983, over a billion doses have been administered worldwide, and in China the rate of childhood infection has fallen from 15 per cent to less than 1 per cent.

I received the hepatitis B vaccine when it was released in Australia in 1984 – just as the AIDS epidemic was gaining momentum. While the current genetically-engineered vaccine is produced in yeast cells and poses absolutely no risk of transmission, the first generation vaccine that I was given was extracted and concentrated from the pooled serum of people who had high levels of hepatitis B antigen in their blood. Since many of these were gay men, there was considerable angst among those who had been vaccinated. I attended a lecture by Ian Gust, who was then also a member of the newly formed AIDS Taskforce. When asked about the vaccine and the risk of AIDS contamination, he went into considerable detail about the way the serum was heat-treated and formalin-inactivated, and how only the non-infectious hepatitis B surface antigen component was left. 'The chance of you catching AIDS from the hepatitis B vaccine is about the same probability of you being kicked to death by a duck', he concluded, leaving me reassured, if somewhat watchful near ponds and lakes.

This is the real epidemic

Once hepatitis A and hepatitis B had been identified and widespread blood-testing of the populations at risk undertaken, it became apparent that there was a third hepatitis virus circulating. Some injecting drug users with chronic hepatitis and cirrhosis of the liver had no evidence of infection with hepatitis B. Furthermore, acute hepatitis was still occurring after blood transfusion, even though the blood had been shown to be clear of the hepatitis B virus. The unknown virus had an incubation period of between two weeks and six months. It is not clear who coined the term, but I suspect Michael Palin or another member of the Monty Python team: the virus that was neither hepatitis A nor hepatitis B became known as hepatitis non-A, non-B.

In the late 1980s, scientists at Chiron, a large US pharmaceutical company, screened several million combinations of gene fragments, looking for one that would react with antibodies found in the blood of laboratory chimpanzees infected with non-A, non-B hepatitis. When they found the nucleotide needle in the DNA haystack in 1989, it was possible to develop an antibody test for what they now renamed hepatitis C. It could be argued that this discovery marked the birth of molecular virology because it would be over ten years before the virus itself could be cultured in the laboratory. Never before had the genetic structure of a pathogen been elucidated without knowing what the bug actually looked like.

Once the hepatitis C antibody tests were available in 1990 it was possible to show that 75 per cent of post-transfusion hepatitis had been due to hepatitis C. Immediately blood banks introduced the test and hundreds of thousands of infections were prevented. When the serum from patients at Fairfield who had been diagnosed with non-A, non-B hepatitis over the previous 20 years was screened by the new test it was confirmed that almost all of them had been infected with hepatitis C.

Before the antibody test came on-line, the number of people infected with hepatitis C had been grossly under-estimated. Hepatitis C, unlike A and B, only rarely causes an illness that is recognised by the patient at the time the infection is acquired –

that is, acute hepatitis. Hepatitis C does its damage slowly and insidiously, with no early warning, and it was only when patients developed cirrhosis or liver cancer that a diagnosis of hepatitis C was suspected. It was soon found that the majority of people who were current injecting drug users were infected with hepatitis C. The longer someone injected, the greater their chance of testing positive for the virus; even baby-boomers who had experimented only briefly with injecting drugs in their youth were discovering that they carried the virus in their blood.

It is estimated that there are 170 million people with hepatitis C around the world, the majority of cases being related to transfusion and injecting drug use. Once the blood supply was secured, injecting drug use became the almost exclusive risk factor for infection, although infected women can transmit the infection to their children at birth, who then usually remain infected for life. Between two-thirds and three-quarters of people who are infected with hepatitis C will go on to develop liver damage, ranging from chronic hepatitis to cirrhosis, and about 8 per cent of these will develop liver cancer. This is a sobering thought for many people in Egypt, where up to 20 per cent of the population is infected with hepatitis C. This is a medical tragedy. The virus is believed to have been transmitted by medically prescribed injections given to the population as part of an eradication campaign against the parasitic disease schistosomiasis carried out from the 1960s to the 1980s.

In Australia at least 280 000 people have contracted hepatitis C – which translates into around 1.3 per cent of the population. Without treatment about 210 000 will stay carriers of the virus for life, 140 000 are likely to develop some degree of liver damage and as many as 28 000 will develop cirrhosis or liver cancer. Compare these numbers with the HIV epidemic in Australia: there have been 28 000 HIV infections since 1983 and 10 000 deaths. The surviving 18 000 patients are likely to have a close to normal life-span if they receive antiviral medication. If I took you around my hospital today I could show you at least half a-dozen patients who are there because of complications caused by hepatitis C infection. It is unlikely that there would be any in-patients with an HIV-related illness. It is hepatitis C that has given us the epidemic we all feared HIV would deliver.

The way that hepatitis C causes disease is nowhere near as varied as HIV. At risk of sounding a little flippant, hepatitis C is a mundane virus – like all the hepatitis viruses it virtually only causes one thing, liver damage, and that translates into a reasonably narrow range of symptoms and signs.

The liver is your body's Big Yellow Taxi, because, as Joni Mitchell says, you don't know what you've got 'til it's gone … The hepatitis C patient may feel tired and out of sorts for many years because the virus causes low-grade inflammation of the liver; the inflammation eventually causes death of liver cells and non-functioning scars are the end-result. Eventually the whole liver becomes one lump of scar tissue – this is cirrhosis – and the patient develops liver failure.

The liver is a producer and a processor. It makes the proteins that help our blood clot. It makes albumin, which stops the blood in our veins from leaking into the surrounding tissues. It processes fats and makes the cholesterol that our nerves need to stay intact. The liver acts as a short-term store of glucose that can be mobilised in minutes when we exercise, and it can make sugars anew when necessary. The liver changes dangerous chemicals and substances into safe ones – it metabolises alcohol into non-intoxicating by-products and breaks down morphine and other drugs. When our liver fails so do we. The body starts to swell, the belly bloats, the eyes go yellow and we lapse in and out of consciousness. Liver failure might be stereotyped but it is an awful fate. There is no drug treatment that can reverse established cirrhosis; the only cure is a liver transplant – and even then the transplanted liver can become infected with hepatitis C. Rewind, replay. The year 2008 was a record one for liver transplants in Australia – 229 were performed and around 45 of these were for people with hepatitis C. That leaves just 27 955 cases of hepatitis C-related cirrhosis to go.

Once you know what a virus looks like, how it reproduces in the host cell and what enzymes it uses, you can design a therapy for it. The basic principles of the life-cycle of HIV were understood within a few years of its discovery and rational drug design led to the production of powerful antiviral agents. There are now also highly active antivirals for hepatitis B that, interestingly, target the same family of enzymes as some of the drugs used against HIV. A single daily pill can now stop the replication of hepatitis B and halt the liver inflammation in over 80 per cent of patients. Unfortunately neither HIV nor hepatitis B is currently curable: once you stop the drugs the virus starts to replicate again. Treatment for hepatitis C, on the other hand, can actually cure the patient of the infection. The catch is that overall only between 50 and 60 per cent of patients respond and the treatment takes six months. Things are getting better, though, and it is likely that within the next ten years cure rates of over 80 per cent will be possible.

Yet, despite these quiet miracles of modern rational drug design, only a very small minority of people with hepatitis B and hepatitis C receive treatment. There were 3500 people treated for hepatitis C in Australia in 2007, which represents around 2 per cent of those who need it. How can this be?

Organise or die

The answer, as always, lies in the epidemiology. The vast majority of new hepatitis C infections occur among injecting drug users. In Australia this group has been well represented on high-level government committees for more than a decade, but its advocacy started a decade after the mobilisation of the political voice of HIV patients. Furthermore, HIV in Australia mainly affected gay men, who came from all strata of society. Many HIV lobbyists were doctors, lawyers, senior public servants and other professionals, and they knew how to play the game in Canberra. Although by no means absent from the professional classes, injecting drug use occurs principally in those who are poor, disadvantaged and at the edges of the society. In the HIV arena, barriers to treatment uptake would be quickly identified and then removed, but similar impediments to hepatitis C treatment stood for many years. It is only in the last five years that it has been possible for a patient to start hepatitis C treatment without first having a liver biopsy. Such is the word on the street about the pain and risk of a biopsy that this requirement frightened many prospective patients away. The need to complete six months of treatment that causes unpleasant side-effects and to demonstrate that you are not still injecting further reduces the rate of treatment uptake.

And if measures to identify and treat people with hepatitis C in Australia have been slow in coming, they have been even slower in the case of those with hepatitis B, where most of those infected belong to ethnic groups who come from countries where the disease is highly prevalent – principally China and nations of southeast Asia. There are around 100 000 people with chronic hepatitis B infection in Australia and the vast majority of these would benefit from treatment. The first specific national hepatitis B strategy appeared in 2009 – 20 years after the first HIV strategy was released. A Rolls-Royce combination of antiviral treatment has been available for the past ten years for those hepatitis B sufferers who are co-infected with HIV, but those who are infected with hepatitis B alone were not able to access the same drugs through the Pharmaceuticals Benefits Scheme (PBS) until 2009.

The outsider may believe that there is an inherent wisdom in the health system – that a group of experts sits above the noise and bustle and makes sensible decisions about the best way to allocate the billions of dollars that are available. To some degree this is so – when a new drug is presented to the government for consideration of approval and subsidy, the relevant committee uses evidence-based principles to determine if the drug is safe, that it works and that it would be cost-effective. Overall, this process works quite well, and it tempers the profit-driven motives of the pharmaceuticals industry. But it is a reactive system – the government responds to applications, it rarely initiates them. It is only when powerful lobbying occurs that it takes a more active role – the fast-tracking of HIV drugs in response to cogent community-based advocacy being a good example of this.

Which medical group 'owns' the disease also matters. In Australia, HIV is managed by infectious diseases physicians, immunologists and 'high-caseload' general practitioners. Hepatitis, on the other hand, is managed mainly by gastroenterologists. The usual cross-specialty rivalries exist between all these groups, and we infectious diseases doctors often suggest that the gastroenterologists don't take the same community-based approach to hepatitis that we took to HIV. It could be argued that the gastroenterologists' insistence over so many years that a liver biopsy was required before starting treatment was an example of the 'excellent being the enemy of the good' – by mandating a meticulous assessment of the stage of each individual patient's liver disease, dozens of other patients were denied the opportunity for treatment. And if you have doubts that medical decisions are made in response to lobbying, consider the fact that the requirement for liver biopsy for hepatitis C was removed from the PBS rules in 2006 but is still in place for hepatitis B.

One of Australia's great public health coups was to introduce needle-exchange before HIV became established in the injecting drug user population. Because we are so used to this approach today, it is easy to forget how radical the proposal was at the time (needle exchange was introduced in New South Wales in 1986 and soon after in Victoria). Here was government taking a cross-eyed view of drugs policy – on the one hand adopting a strong anti-drugs stance in respect of law enforcement and importation control, on the other recognising the need for 'harm-minimisation' measures to limit the long-term consequences of injecting drug use. Today less than 1 per cent of current injecting drug users in Australia have HIV, compared to 12 per cent in China, 16 per cent in the USA and a staggering 37 per cent in Russia.

So, if needle and syringe programs were so effective in keeping HIV out of the injecting drug user population, why is it that nearly 60 per cent of current Australian injecting drug users have hepatitis C? Again, it's the epidemiology. HIV is less transmissible that hepatitis C by a factor of about ten, and when the programs were introduced HIV was rare among Australian injecting drug users. Needle exchange reduces needle sharing but does not eliminate it: for HIV the reduction in sharing rates was enough to prevent the infection from becoming endemic, but to have an effect on the transmission of hepatitis C, which was already endemic, it would have required complete cessation of needle sharing. It is the difference between a game of Russian roulette when five chambers of the gun are loaded (hepatitis C) and one in which most pistols don't even have one chamber loaded (HIV). By the time needle exchange was introduced in parts of Europe and the USA it was too late: HIV was by then common among injecting drug users. Timing in public health is everything.

More viral arrivals

A tour of viral hepatitis is not, I'm afraid to say, quite as easy as ABC. In 1980 a hepatitis virus that can only infect the liver of someone who already has hepatitis B was discovered. It was originally called delta hepatitis, but once hepatitis C was named in 1989, it became hepatitis D. Co-infection with hepatitis D can worsen the liver damage already being caused by hepatitis B. The good news is that vaccination against B protects you against D as well. Hepatitis D is very uncommon in the developed world except among injecting drug users, so probably goes undiagnosed in many instances. A much more important virus is hepatitis E, which, while very rare in developed countries, has been the cause of large outbreaks of hepatitis in the developing world. It behaves like hepatitis A – it has a similar incubation period and causes the same kind of illness. The major difference is that hepatitis E has a very high mortality rate in pregnant women – up to 20 per cent of whom die of liver failure if they are infected during the third trimester. A vaccine is in the late stages of development. Hepatitis G is related to hepatitis C, but it is a virus looking for a disease. Up to 2 per cent of the population carry it but it does not appear to cause any ill-effects. There are no routine tests available to diagnose it.

A, B, C, D, E, G. But what about F? I hear you ask. In the 1990s evidence of a toga virus which caused hepatitis was published by French researchers. It was originally called hepatitis F. But the research findings could not be reproduced and are now discredited. One afternoon I finished my lecture on hepatitis with this fact – at which point one of my students, known for his love of profanity, commented, 'Thank God, the end of F in hepatitis' … which, for the time being at least, it is.

15

Sleepers, wake

Neisseria meningitidis – a Gram-negative bacterium that forms
pairs and lives within white blood cells. Although
N. meningitidis can produce one of the most feared of human
diseases – meningococcal meningitis – it is present in the throat
of about 10 per cent of well young people. Only a tiny minority
of these infected individuals develop meningococcal disease –
for the rest, the organism peacefully co-exists with them and
causes no harm. It is closely related to the bacterium that causes
gonorrhoea.

'There are seeds of self-destruction in all of us that will bear only
unhappiness if allowed to grow.' (from *Wake up and Live*, by
Dorothea Brande, 1893–1948)

Depending on the company and my mood, I may tell dinner
party companions that I am a specialist in infectious diseases
rather than a sexual health doctor. Sometimes I lead with the
latter as a device to avoid having talk to the person who first
engaged me in conversation; in other cases it can be the beginning of a beautiful relationship. Usually though, I opt for the
former, safer, choice and the reply is often something like: 'But
why would you choose Canberra? There can't be many infectious
diseases in Canberra'. Au contraire, my dear friend, au contraire.

One of the fundamental achievements of evolution has been the adaptation of humans to cope with the invisible zoo of micro-organisms that coat their skin, live in the food and water that they consume, and float in the air that they breathe. Although we have names for the thousands that are known to cause disease, there are anonymous millions that live in the environment, pass through our gastro-intestinal tracts and cause no harm. Many of the more malign bacteria that *do* cause disease can also peacefully co-exist with us – this is called colonisation. The promotion of domestic antibacterial products for the kitchen and bathroom supports a belief in the public's mind that the enemy is always at the gates – that a dirty dishcloth is the modern day equivalent of the smallpox-encrusted blanket. There is a kernel of truth in this, but, in the developed world at least, more often the enemy is actually within. Most of us already carry the seeds of our own destruction, silently drawing the minute amount of nutrients that they need from our mucous membranes (throat, nose or vagina), but causing no harm, just trying to get on with their usually asexual and, I would have to say, boring little lives. But sometimes, like KGB sleeper agents planted in the suburbs of middle England in the 1950s waiting for the revolution, a coded message is sent, the coloniser is activated, and neighbour changes into assassin.

Not a bit like on the television

I had just finished my Saturday morning ward round and was sitting in my car contemplating what I would do with the rest of the day when my phone rang. It was a general practitioner who provided services to one of the regional boarding schools ringing for advice. I knew him quite well and I could immediately sense from his voice that something terrible had happened. One of the senior students at the school hadn't appeared at breakfast and a few hours later had been found dead in his room by another student. He had been unwell with the flu the day before and had seen one of the doctor's partners. The police had been called and they had immediately noticed that the young man was covered in a purple rash. 'It's bloody awful. This has got to be meningococcal disease', the GP said. 'My partner is a mess because he feels responsible and I've got to decide what to do with the rest of the school.'

I told him that I would call the public health unit, which would start to co-ordinate a response, and that I would examine the body when it was transferred to the city mortuary to confirm the diagnosis. I would need microbiological evidence, but we would want to give the public health team advice as soon as possible.

There are things that no parent should see, and I would be a little uncomfortable relating the next part of the story if there wasn't a point to it. The post-1945 generations have, in the main, been spared first-hand experience of the sights and sounds of death, and it is not surprising that we are intrigued by its fictional depiction. The popularity of forensic investigation dramas has spawned a special-effects industry that creates uncannily life-like, or more correctly, death-like, mannequins. Every time I turn on the television, it seems, I am exposed to actors up to their elbows in the body cavity of what looks like a real person. It is easy to believe, therefore, that we have become inured to the blood and gore of death, that the real thing would be just like the TV. It isn't. I have seen and examined dozens of dead bodies, but I still dread the sight of a human on a mortuary slab. It is a little easier when you don't know the person, or they are old and the death was expected. But when you are confronted by the body of a 17 year old, one's internal composure weakens and the hardened doctor becomes a vulnerable father. It is crucial to keep this effect to yourself: the last thing that a traumatised family needs is a distraught medical attendant.

I drove to the forensic centre, which was hidden in a then

unpopulated part of town near to the lake. I entered the mortuary room, greeted the attendant and asked to examine the body. ('The body' – for that was what a young man had become now, and for the moment I would stay with this self-protective deceit.) I tried to avoid looking at the face and eyes. I could see a rash on the arms, legs and trunk. They had the appearance of vivid bruises – the typical rash of meningococcal sepsis. I asked the mortuary attendant to collect a sample of blood and courier it to our microbiology laboratory. One of our technicians would look at a stained slide of the blood under a microscope. There are virtually no other infections where this technique can show the presence of bacteria – usually you have to amplify the number of organisms by culturing them in the laboratory for at least 12, and usually 24 to 48 hours. But in a small proportion of cases of meningococcal disease you can see the bacteria in the blood sample itself without needing to resort to culture.

Putting the story together with the physical findings, I was satisfied that the clinical diagnosis was meningococcal septicaemia. Rarely, other infections can cause almost identical symptoms to what I had seen on the young man, but I had enough information now to advise the public health unit that they should start tracing his contacts.

The mantle of most feared disease

Neisseria meningitidis is one of the most powerful bacterial pathogens that infect humans. It grows rapidly in both the laboratory and in the humans it infects – it can double its numbers within hours. The different strains of the bacterium are divided according to the types of antigens that they have on their surface – these can be detected in the laboratory by incubating the culture with a panel of antibodies. Most human disease is caused by serogroups A, B or C. The A serogroup is associated with epidemics of meningococcal disease in the 'meningitis belt' of sub-Saharan Africa, but it occasionally causes disease in the developed world as well. Serogroups B and C are responsible for most of the cases that occur in the West. Infection usually strikes in early childhood or in adolescence/young adulthood, but people of any age can get it.

The bacterium is almost always sensitive to penicillin, but this is no cause for comfort – infection with bacteria that are treatable with the simplest antibiotics can still cause terrible disease and rapidly progress to death. The clinical manifestations of meningococcal disease lie along a spectrum ranging from colonisation of the throat, which causes no ill-effects, to a mild infection causing a scattered rash, arthritis and fever, to meningitis (an infection of the covering of the brain), to overwhelming sepsis – which results in kidney, lung and heart failure, and ultimately death. Meningococcal disease is a frightening condition for parents and for doctors. While the majority of young people with the disease will recover, a significant proportion of them will suffer serious complications. The collapse of the circulation can lead to loss of blood supply to the arms and legs, and the amputation of fingers, toes and even limbs is not an uncommon consequence.

Now that the vaccine-preventable diseases that scared previous generations of parents have almost disappeared – for example, diphtheria, measles, whooping cough, polio and tetanus – meningococcal disease has taken on the mantle of most-feared disease. When a case is reported in the press, parents panic about their children attending group activities and sharing drink bottles at school. However, here is an important but little known fact: if the throats of all first-year university students were swabbed, *N. meningitidis* would be found in about 10 per cent of them, yet it would be rare to find a case of meningococcal illness in any of them. The majority of people will have encountered the organism during their life, but it is almost always held in check by the immune system: the bug just sits there causing no harm whatsoever.

Although we don't classify these bacteria as such, what I am describing is essentially a host–parasite relationship: a potentially deadly game of microbiological Mexican stand-off – don't hurt me, I won't hurt you. The bacterium gains because it can only survive in humans – becoming virulent and causing death is, in effect, a biological dead-end for it. Sometimes, however, this balance is upset: a change in the proteins on the surface of the bacterium may occur and the circulating strain takes on a greater ability to cause invasive disease. Then, when the bug is transferred to another person through kissing or other means of fluid transfer, it may evade the immune response and spread to the outer part of the brain, causing headache, neck stiffness, fever and a rash – meningococcal meningitis. Again, it is not widely appreciated that it is better to have this manifestation of meningococcal disease than meningococcal septicaemia, where the immune system has not been able to hold the disease within the central nervous system and it has spread throughout the body. The mortality from meningococcal meningitis is around 5 per cent, but is just over twice that, about 11 per cent, for meningococcal septicaemia.

When a young person contracts meningococcal disease in a school or other educational setting we worry that a cluster (handful) of cases will follow, or worse, a larger outbreak. Such events are rare today in Australia but used to be common in boarding schools and military barracks. Most cases today are what is known as sporadic, and we don't see any more infections related to the original one (known as the index case). However, you can't tell from the outset what is going to happen, and the accepted practice is to find the people who have been in close contact with the index case and, if they meet certain criteria, to offer them what is known as antibiotic prophylaxis. All household contacts are offered this as a matter of course, but the guidelines say that the only other people who should receive antibiotics are those who have had intimate contact with the victim or shared the same space as them for four hours or more. The panic and fear that surround a case of meningococcal disease make it difficult to adhere to these guidelines because worried parents ask you, sometimes implore you, to give their children prophylaxis. This is understandable, and many people used to the liberal prescription of antibiotics for minor complaints are confused and even annoyed when we recommend against prophylaxis. Less understandable is when medical staff ask for prophylaxis when it is not indicated – they should know better, but their behaviour supports my hypothesis about what drives infection control *(see chapter 8)*. Most people, many doctors included, believe that the reason for prescribing the antibiotics is to prevent the contacts from developing meningococcal disease. In fact, the principal rationale for their use is to eradicate the meningococcus from the throat of contacts and thus stop them from transmitting the bacterium to other susceptible individuals.

There are very few bacteria that can kill an otherwise fit and well young person in such a short time (another is *Streptococcus pneumoniae*, or pneumococcus) and it is no wonder that the population is frightened of meningococcal disease and doctors dread mis-diagnosing it. But the reality is that a GP is unlikely to ever see a case. Between 300 and 400 people develop meningococcal sepsis each year in Australia, and a significant number of these will go straight to hospital and not be seen in general practice. Our unit ran a program where GPs could accompany us on our main ward round of the week. One of the best GPs in town, a man with over 25 years clinical experience, attended a round and I took him to see a young man on the ward who was recovering from meningococcal sepsis. The patient still had the characteristic rash on his arms and legs. The GP was thrilled to have the opportunity to look at the patient because he had never before seen anyone with the rash.

New Zealand has been experiencing an epidemic of meningococcal disease over the past two decades, caused mainly by one serotype of the germ, and peaking at an average of 400 cases a year over the two years 2002 and 2003 – though only about 30 deaths were recorded over this peak period. This is another medical paradox – the more common a potentially lethal condition in a population, the more alert doctors are to it and the more likely you are to receive appropriate and early treatment. In a population where the incidence of the disease is lower, a doctor is more likely to miss the diagnosis when a patient with the infection is seen. Although comparisons are problematic, it appears that the death rate in New Zealand from meningococcal disease was actually lower during its epidemic than in Australia over the same period. One possible explanation for this is that the protocols for the early administration of antibiotics are adhered to better in New Zealand than they are in Australia.

All young people in Australia are now offered conjugated meningococcal vaccine, but this is only protective against the C serotype of the bacterium. (It was the B serotype that was responsible for the outbreak of meningococcal disease in New Zealand, cases of which have dropped dramatically over recent years, partly due to the local development of a vaccine against the serotype.) There is a vaccine which covers A, C and some of the other serotypes, but it is not very potent. Wherever the conjugated type C vaccine has been rolled out, the number of cases of meningococcal disease falls, but until a vaccine that protects against the three main serotypes is developed the disease will continue to kill people of all ages regardless of the degree of vigilance of the medical system.

The miasma of fear

The GP was on the phone again. The school principal was pushing for every boarder in the school to receive prophylaxis. I could understand his desire to pursue this but I knew of a similar circumstance in another institutional setting where several hundred people had received prophylaxis, almost all of them outside of the guideline recommendations. One person, who didn't meet the criteria, had developed anaphylaxis to the antibiotic administered, collapsed in the doctor's surgery and had to be resuscitated. I told the GP my views and he subsequently received the same advice from the public health unit. But I knew he would have a hard time convincing the school that not everyone needed prophylaxis, and I knew that in the miasma of fear that surrounds such events it is impossible to always adhere to evidence-based decision making. I also knew that there was another person to consider in this tragedy – the doctor who had seen the student the day before his death; I asked the GP on the phone how his colleague was.

'Terrible', he said, 'absolutely shattered'. They always are, I thought to myself, for this is the way it usually goes.

A few weeks later I learnt that 24 hours before he died the student had gone to the school nurse with a fever and a mild headache. She had taken him to the GP surgery, where the doctor on duty for urgent cases saw him. There was a lot of viral illness around at the time; many other students from the school had been unwell with a runny nose, low-grade fever and a general flu-like illness. The young man didn't look that unwell, there were no specific findings when the doctor examined him, and, in particular, there was no rash anywhere on his body. He advised the patient to have the next day off school, to take paracetamol and to keep up his fluid intake. The student was one of a dozen young people the GP had seen that day with similar symptoms. The doctor didn't give the student another thought until he received a phone call from the police the following day. At some stage over the 12 hours following his visit to the surgery, the young man had deteriorated and, alone in his bedroom overnight, would have died a lonely death.

There would be a coronial inquest and the recommendation would almost certainly be that doctors and nurses should be more aware of the illness, and parents and teachers should learn to recognise the early warning signs. This is reasonable advice and I can understand the sentiment, but while it is in its early stages it is incredibly difficult to differentiate meningococcal disease from other less serious conditions, and you can't admit every young person with a fever to hospital. Without the rash it is extremely hard to make the diagnosis – and sometimes the rash can appear only hours before the patient dies. A worrying point for public health education is that the patients who are most likely to die from meningococcal infection will not have neck stiffness, which is most commonly perceived to be an indicator of the disease. A series of cases from the UK showed that in addition to fever and the patient feeling unwell, the most important clinical sign for a doctor to recognise in early meningococcal sepsis is severe pain in the muscles of the legs.

Days and then weeks passed and, as we expected, there were no more cases linked to the school. It is impossible to know if the prophylaxis was responsible for the absence of any new cases. While it would be very difficult to abandon this long-established public health intervention, most authorities feel that antibiotics play only a small part in the prevention of outbreaks. For some reason, this unfortunate young man had contracted a strain of meningococcus that had evaded his immune system. There were probably hundreds of his friends and schoolmates who had acquired, accommodated and eradicated the bug from their systems without suffering any ill-effects. The strain that the student who died contracted obviously wasn't particularly virulent or other cases would have arisen. We will never know why he was affected and others were spared.

After I have had a bad week at work I start to remember my dreams again. In the nights that followed I found myself hovering over the city, as if in a film. I start in the clouded sky and then track in so that I am close enough to see the life going on in individual houses. The silent silhouettes of domestic activity are visible to my camera eye as I float past the windows, but I am hidden to the occupants within. I move out again to take in the whole expanse of the population below. Suddenly I swoop down to one home and, in the calm logic of the dream, I realise that I am Death and that this is the address of the child that I have chosen. A cold fear grips me because I know that if I can only wake up I will spare this family. Again and again I awaken into the same dream. But now the phone by my bed is vibrating and I know that I can climb the ascending tone of its ring into wakefulness. It is the hospital, of course, and they are so, so wrong to apologise for waking me.

'Just putting you through to the emergency department, doctor'.

I pray that someone very old is dying.

Glossary

Acute A disease or condition that has a short time course from onset to recovery– for example, acute hepatitis. A common cause of miscommunication between the doctor and patient; many acute conditions are serious but this is not always the case. See also *chronic*.

Aetiology The cause or origin of a disease

Aerobic Literally 'air life'. Organisms that require oxygen to multiply are called aerobes.

Agar plate Circular plastic dish containing agar, a jelly-like substance derived from algae and seaweed. The agar may contain additional nutrients to allow the growth of the target bacteria, and antibiotics and other suppressants to inhibit the overgrowth of non-pathogens.

Anaerobic Literally 'without air life' . Organisms that multiply in the absence of oxygen are called anaerobes.

Aniline dye An organic (i.e. carbon-containing) compound discovered in the 1850s and originally used in the dye industry. Sulfonamide antibiotics are derived from aniline dyes.

Antibiotic Coined in 1942 by the US microbiologist Selman Waksman (discoverer of the anti-TB drug streptomycin) to describe a substance produced by a micro-organism that kills or inhibits the growth of bacteria. This strict definition would exclude synthetic compounds such as sulphonamides and most modern antibacterial drugs. Today antibiotic refers to any compound with activity against bacteria and fungi. See also, *sulphur drug*.

Antibody A protein that circulates in the blood and other bodily fluids to neutralise material foreign to the body – for example, a *bacterium* or *virus*.

Antigen Literally 'that which produces an *antibody*'. Virtually any molecule or substance can be an antigen – for example, pollens, bacteria, viruses and other pathogens.

Antigenic drift Minor changes in the antigens on the surface of an influenza virus due to random mutations that occur as the *virus* replicates.

Antigenic shift A major change in the structure of an influenza virus that occurs when the genetic material of two separate organisms re-assort to form a new virus. Antigenic shift may result in a flu *pandemic*. See also, *re-assortment*.

Antiretroviral A drug which inhibits the multiplication of a *retrovirus* such as *HIV*.

Bacterium A single-celled micro-organism that lacks a nucleus. Most bacteria are free- living in the environment but some can only survive in humans and other higher animals.

Base pair DNA is composed of molecules called bases: adenine (A), cytosine (C), guanine (G) and thymine (T), which comprise the genetic codes of all living things. A binds with T and G binds with C to form base pairs to form the double-stranded helix of *DNA*.

Campylobacter A *Gram-negative* bacterium that is one of the commonest bacterial causes of food poisoning.

CDC Centers for Disease Control and Prevention, in Atlanta, Georgia. The peak institution for identifying and controlling communicable diseases in the USA.

Capillary The smallest blood vessels in the human body. These tiny tubes carry oxygen and other nutrients to the tissues.

Chronic A disease or condition that has a protracted time course from its onset– for example, emphysema, one of the conditions that comprises chronic obstructive pulmonary disease. Often incorrectly used by non-medical people to imply severity. See also, *acute*.

Coloniser An organism that can be found in a site in the human body – for example, the throat, vagina or skin – but which may be causing no disease. Colonisers have the potential to cause invasive disease.

DNA Deoxyribonucleic acid – a compound, found in almost all living things, that contains the genetic material necessary for inheritance of characteristics and the organisation and function of cells. See also, *base pair*.

Endemic A disease which is always present in a population.

Family A grouping of organisms containing (usually) more than one *genus*. See also *taxonomy*.

Fungus A family of organisms that includes yeasts and moulds. Most are not pathogens but a small number cause human illness ranging from mild conditions such as tinea to serious life-threatening disease – for example, candida blood poisoning.

Genus A grouping of (usually) several species of organisms sharing common characteristics. A taxonomic rank between *family* and *species*. See also *taxonomy*.

Gram positive/negative A simple staining technique that was first described by the Danish pathologist Hans Christian Gram in 1884 and is still the most important first step in bacterial identification in the modern microbiological laboratory. A bacterium is Gram positive if it appears purple and Gram negative if pink under the microscope.

Guillain-Barré syndrome Inflammation of the peripheral nerves that usually produces 'ascending paralysis' – that is, progressive weakness that starts at the feet and works its way up the body. The condition can follow an infection such as *campylobacter* food poisoning or influenza.

Haemorrhagic fever A disease characterised by fever and bleeding, with a high mortality. It is caused by several viruses – for example, Marburg, Ebola, Hantavirus – which are confined to Africa and South America.

HIV Human immunodeficiency virus.

Immunosuppression An impairment in the ability to fight infection due to a deficiency in one or more components of the immune system. Most immunosuppression in the developed world is a complication of the treatments for cancer and autoimmune diseases (such as rheumatoid arthritis) and secondary to the drugs used to prevent rejection following organ transplantation. The major cause in the developing world is *HIV* infection.

Iron lung A container that housed patients with polio who had lost the function of the muscles needed for respiration. The patient would lie with only their head outside the iron lung with an airtight seal at their neck. The pressure inside would be cyclically raised and lowered to create a negative pressure which would passively draw in air through the patient's mouth. The 'iron lungs' at Fairfield Hospital were constructed of wood.

Lumen The inside of a hollow organ such as the large or small intestine.

Neoplasm Literally 'new formation'; can refer to any tumour or cancer.

Nucleotide Molecules that join together to form the structure of *DNA* and *RNA*.

Pandemic An epidemic that affects the entire world. From the Greek, meaning 'all people'.

Parasite From the Latin, 'one who eats at the table of another'. An organism that lives in or on another and benefits at the cost of the other organism. All pathogens are technically parasites but traditionally the term has been confined to the endoparasites and ectoparasites. Worms, such as hookworm, and protozoa, such as malaria, are endoparasites. *Sarcoptes scabiei* (the cause of scabies) and *Pediculus humanis capitis* (the cause of head lice) are examples of ectoparasites.

Pathogen Any micro-organism that is known to cause disease. Only a tiny proportion of the known bacteria, viruses and fungi and other micro-organisms are human pathogens.

Peritoneal cavity A potential space inside the abdomen formed by the membrane (peritoneum) which lines the abdominal cavity.

Prophylaxis The use of an antibiotic or antiviral agent to reduce the chance of someone who has been exposed to a *pathogen* becoming infected.

Protozoan A micro-organism whose genetic material is contained within a nucleus, making it a more complex life-form than a *bacterium*.

Pyrexia Fever. Defined as a temperature greater than 37.5 degrees Celsius. Fever is usually an indicator of infection but it can occur in association with non-infectious conditions such as cancer and auto-immune disease.

Re-assortment The mixing of genetic material from different viruses to produce a new strain. Also known as recombination.

RNA Ribonucleic acid. A chain of *nucleotides* that mediates protein synthesis and regulates the function of cells. The genetic information of many viruses is encoded as RNA.

Retrovirus An *RNA* virus that incorporates its genetic material into the *DNA* of the cells that it infects – for example *HIV*.

SARS Severe Acute Respiratory Syndrome.

Serum The liquid part of blood that has had the red blood cells separated out by spinning at high speed in a centrifuge. The remaining clear yellowish liquid contains antibodies, hormones, proteins, glucose and mineral ions.

Sero-positive/negative The presence or absence in the serum of antibodies to a particular pathogen or condition.

Species A grouping of organisms capable of exchanging genetic material or interbreeding. The lowest taxonomic rank. See also *taxonomy*.

Sulphur drug Synthetic antibacterial compounds that possess a sulphur-containing group called sulphonamide.

Taxonomy The science of the classification of organisms according to shared characteristics.

Toxoid A toxin which has been chemically changed to weaken its original toxicity. Toxoids are used to vaccinate against tetanus and diphtheria.

Virus An infectious agent that can only reproduce inside the living cells of another organism. Viruses are composed of genetic material – either *DNA* or *RNA* – a protein coat and sometimes a lipid (fatty) envelope. Viruses can infect plants, animals and other micro-organisms such as bacteria.

WHO World Health Organization.

Window period The time between infection with a pathogen and the appearance of antibodies against it in the *serum*.

Acknowledgments

I am indebted to a number of people for their comments and support.

My special thanks to Ivan Bastian, Sophie Bertram, Sean Bowden, Greg Clarke, Peter Collignon, Kit Fairley, Tom Faunce, Merryn Hare, Jenny Hurley, Karina Kennedy, Denise Kraus, Sarah Martin, Malcolm McDonald, Sanjaya Senanayake, Francis Sullivan, Ashwin Swaminathan, Leon Tetlow and Ashley Watson. I am grateful to all the staff of UNSW Press, in particular Heather Champion, who was my original champion, Heather Cam for her overall guidance and Jane McCredie, who showed me how to restructure the text to create a more coherent book and whose support has been invaluable. My wonderful copy editor, Neil Thomson, gently helped me to reshape and hone my arguments, and on several occasions made me realise that my prose was indeed deathless – zombie-like, that is.

The responsibility for any errors and omissions remain mine alone.

Allen Yung has been the role model for a generation of Australian infectious diseases physicians – teacher, mentor, philosopher, diagnostician and humanitarian – and although he doesn't appear in this book, he is a silent presence in most, if not all, of the stories presented here.

Brian Kennedy, by dint of an inscription in a book he gave

me as a birthday present, finally motivated me to take the time to collect these stories. Much earlier, Noelene Gore encouraged a tired young resident to take up writing again – it only took 20 years, Noelene!

The other sexually transmitted beings in my life, my children, Madeleine, Joshua and Lucy, have put up with their father's preoccupation with this book (as well as a lifetime of unusual dinner conversation) and I thank them for occasionally giving me a hint of encouragement. My wife, Philippa Keating, remains my closest and favourite critic – hard but fair – although she did allow me to overhear two or three chuckles as she read the manuscript in bed at night.

Index to pathogens and diseases